ABOUT THE AUTHORS

MELISSA BROOKS is a sociology graduate from the University of Durham. She has worked for many years in publishing before concentrating on women's health as a freelance editor and writer. She co-wrote with Dr Anna Flynn *A Manual of Natural Family Planning* (Unwin Hyman, 1985).

MICHAEL ROGERS, MRCOG, FRCS read medicine at the University of Birmingham. He is a member of the Royal College of Obstetricians and a Fellow of the Royal College of Physicians and Surgeons of Glasgow. He is currently Senior Lecturer in Obstetrics and Gynaecology at the Chinese University of Hong Kong.

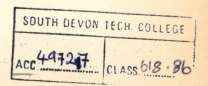

CAESAREAN BIRTH

A PRACTICAL GUIDE

MELISSA BROOKS
WITH DR MICHAEL ROGERS

An OPTIMA book

First published in 1989 by
Macdonald Optima, a division of
Macdonald & Co. (Publishers) Ltd

A member of Maxwell Pergamon Publishing Corporation plc

British Library Cataloguing in Publication Data
Brooks, Melissa
    Caesarean birth.
    1. Childbirth.   Caesarean section. — For
    parents
    I. Title   II. Rogers, Michael
    618.8'6'0240431

    ISBN 0-356-15847-0

Macdonald & Co. (Publishers) Ltd
66-73 Shoe Lane
London EC4P 4AB

Typeset in Century Schoolbook by Leaper & Gard, Bristol

Printed and bound in Great Britain by
The Guernsey Press Co. Ltd., Guernsey, Channel Islands.

CONTENTS

ACKNOWLEDGEMENTS

The publishers would like to thank Jane Bown/
The Observer; Anthea Sieveking/Vision International;
and Camilla Jessel for the photographs.

INTRODUCTION

All mothers-to-be look forward to an uncomplicated, relaxed pregnancy and a natural 'normal' birth. And there is plenty of information available today to help prospective parents understand what happens during pregnancy and what to expect at the birth of their child — scores of books are published on the topic every year, leaflets distributed, guidance and counselling supplied by antenatal clinics. Yet more often than not there is either no reference at all or only a passing comment on birth by caesarean section — and this despite the fact that one in nine women who go into hospital for the birth of their baby will have a caesarean delivery. Sheila Kitzinger, one of Britain's leading experts on birth matters, makes only one reference to caesarean section in her book *The Experience of Childbirth* (Penguin), and that is in the last appendix to the book. Is this meant to imply that all those women whose babies are born by caesarean section do not experience childbirth, that it is nothing more than a medical procedure?

In my personal experience of caesarean birth this was far from the case. An ultrasound scan at 20 weeks of pregnancy had shown that the placenta was so low down on the uterine wall that it partially blocked the birth canal. My consultant told me that the risks to the baby and to me of a normal delivery were too great to contemplate and that a casearean section would need to be performed. Initially I felt very depressed, but as the life-saving aspects of the proposed operation began to sink in I started to feel extremely grateful that modern medicine could offer the chance to save my baby. I decided to find out everything I could about what was involved, what happened during the operation, what choices about my maternity care were still open to me, the best ways to aid recovery afterwards, so that I could approach this type of birth positively. This was the first stumbling block, for search as I might I discovered that there was a complete dearth of useful material on the subject.

The second obstacle was the attitude of other people. When I told the women at the birth classes I had been attending that a caesarean section had been recommended, their initial display of sympathy was quickly replaced by comments such as 'Well, at least you can do it the easy way' and 'You won't need to bother to come any more if you do not need to find out about being in labour.' It was as if a caesarean birth simply didn't count as birth at all.

But I could feel my baby kicking inside me and I had heard her heartbeat, and seen her little limbs waving on the hazy picture of the ultrasound screen. I knew my baby was going to be *born*, even if we did need some help on the way. On the morning of 15 July 1985 I was wheeled into the theatre at St Bartholomew's Hospital in London with James, almost unrecognisable in theatre gown and hat, by my side. I had opted for an epidural anaesthetic so I could be awake to witness the birth of my baby. Ten minutes after the start of the operation, a pair of feet were waved over the screen across my chest to be met by a cheer from the theatre staff. Two minutes later we were handed our baby girl to cuddle and welcome into the world. It was a moment neither of us will ever forget and which stills bring tears to our eyes every time we recall the occasion.

My own experience of childbirth by caesarean section made me determined that caesarean mothers should be offered a better deal. The aim of this book is to make at least one small step in that direction. It is not a discussion about the 'political' implications of the growing number of caesarean sections performed in this country — there are other arenas for that particular debate — but an attempt to provide down-to-earth, practical, reliable information for women who are either going to have or have had a caesarean birth, so they can make the most of their experiences. Much of the advice comes from women who have themselves experienced and coped with this type of delivery, as well as from the professionals in the field. The guiding premise of the whole book is that caesarean birth, as with any other birth, is the joyful beginning of a new life and can, if approached with confidence and knowledge, be a truly rewarding experience of birth.

I have referred to the baby as 'she' throughout the book for practical, sexist and personal reasons: in practical terms it is very cumbersome for the reader if the page is peppered with the phrase 'he or she'; in sexist terms, boys always hog the limelight so why shouldn't the girls have a go; and in personal terms my own baby is a girl.

Many people have helped me during the writing of this book, though perhaps the biggest thank you should go to all the women who wrote to me telling me about their experiences and offering their tips and advice — it is largely their voices that sound in the following pages. My grateful thanks also go to Dr Michael Rogers, for sharing his vast experience and knowledge; to Chloe Fisher, Senior Midwife, Community Midwives at the John Radcliffe Hospital in Oxford, who shared with me the findings of her recent research with colleague Dr Michael Woolridge, Research Fellow in Child Health at Bristol University which formed the basis of the material in Chapter 7; and to Deirdre Mackay MCSP for supplying invaluable advice and information for Chapter 9.

I would also like to thank Harriet Griffey, without whose patience, guidance and sheer faith there never would have been a book; Margarett, who looked after my little girl so happily while I toiled over the word processor; James, for his unquestioning support and encouragement; and finally Chloe for giving me the reason to write in the first place.

Melissa Brooks

1
WHY A CAESAREAN BIRTH?

For the majority of women, childbirth is — physiologically at least — a straightforward natural process, with labour starting spontaneously and being followed by a normal vaginal delivery. For about one in nine women, however, this natural process either fails to happen or has to be interrupted and the baby delivered by caesarean section, a procedure whereby the baby is delivered through an incision in the mother's abdomen. If you happen to be one of these women, then the most immediate questions in your mind will be 'Why? Why did it have to happen? What went wrong?'

The medical indications for a caesarean delivery are numerous and some of them will be outlined in the following pages. If you have had an emergency caesarean delivery or have just been told that a planned caesarean is recommended, one of the first things you should do is try and find exactly why a caesarean was or is necessary in your case. Obviously the first person to ask is your doctor. Hopefully the information in this chapter will help too, but it is your doctor who is in the best position to provide you with the details of your specific case and the reasons that led him or her to consider such a course of action. So talk it through with your doctor — before the event if it is to be an elective caesarean, afterwards if it was done as an emergency — and don't be afraid to voice all the 'whys' that are in your mind.

Understanding the reasons why your baby needed to be delivered by caesarean section is one of the most positive steps towards coming to terms with what has happened and seeing it, not as a failure on your part — a feeling many caesarean mothers express — or wilful interference on the part of the medical profession, but as a procedure that may have saved your baby's life and possibly your's.

It all happened so quickly. My husband was asked to get me to sign a piece of paper, nurses were running around and I was whisked off to theatre. The next thing I knew was hearing Adrian's voice floating through the fog, saying 'She's lovely: she's fine.' I just felt desperately cheated and unable to take anything in. Later the doctor came round to see us and explained that the baby had been the wrong way up so that her foot had come down first — she was trying to do the splits! It was because the baby was so distressed that they had moved fast. As I looked at our little girl lying in her hospital crib by my bed, I realised we had been terribly lucky. We could have lost her.

Mary

AN HISTORICAL NOTE

The frequency with which obstetricians resort to caesarean section has varied considerably over the last few decades, and even today it differs between hospitals. These differences reflect changes in both the way doctors approach the 'management' of childbirth and in women's attitudes towards delivery by this method. The purpose of this book is not to discuss the implications of the number of caesareans performed in British hospitals and whether or not too many such operations are performed too willingly by the medical profession, but simply to provide practical information to help women whose babies are delivered this way. However, a glance at the historical trends can provide a useful insight.

In the 1950s caesarean section was usually considered only as a last resort when all attempts at a vaginal delivery had failed. The only exceptions to this were those caesareans performed where it was known in advance that a vaginal delivery was not possible, for example because of placenta praevia, or because the baby was lying transversely across the uterus (see pp. 15–18).

However, during the 1960s and 1970s caesarean section rates rose dramatically, from less than 5 per cent to as high as 30 per cent in some hospitals. This increase occurred for a number of reasons: anaesthetics had become much safer and doctors wanted to try and reduce the high (relative to present) perinatal mortality figures (this is measured by taking the number of stillbirths and deaths in the first week of life for every 1,000 deliveries); while at the same time new technology had been developed which enabled doctors to assess the health of the baby while it was still in the uterus.

In the early 1970s the caesarean rates peaked. This coincided with a time when the rate of induction of labour reached an astonishing 50 per cent in some hospitals, with few women being allowed to go beyond their expected date of confinement. Yet the methods of induction available at this time were crude and had unpredictable results, with the consequence that many 'unnecessary' caesarean sections were performed.

Fortunately both medical policy and technology have changed since then. More sophisticated and hence more accurate methods of monitoring the baby in the womb have been developed, induction rates have dropped dramatically and the techniques of induction themselves have been refined, leading to far fewer failed inductions. Consequently the caesarean section rate in most hospitals has now fallen to around 10 per cent.

WHY DO A CAESAREAN SECTION?

Your obstetrician will recommend a caesarean delivery if he or she believes that the dangers to you or the baby, or to both of you, of allowing the natural processes to continue significantly outweigh the dangers of caesarean birth.

In most instances where caesarean delivery is recommended, the indications for such a course of action are clear and not open to debate; faced with the same situation, any doctor would make the same recommendation. Occasionally, however, situations arise where opinion does play a part, where one doctor might recommend a caesarean delivery while another might not. One such situation involves the management of breech presentation (when the baby is lying bottom down in the uterus instead of the usual head down or cephalic presentation — see pp. 18–21). Some doctors feel that, particularly for first-time mothers, the risks attached to trying to deliver a breech presentation baby vaginally are too great and would always recommend a caesarean delivery in such cases; other doctors think that in selected cases it is better to let the woman try to deliver vaginally and only if she or the baby gets into difficulties do an emergency caesarean. If you have been recommended a caesarean section on the grounds of a breech presentation, talk it through thoroughly with your doctor so you understand his or her reasoning for doing the operation.

If for any reason you are dissatisfied with the explanation offered as to why a caesarean delivery is deemed necessary, you are free to seek a second opinion. Equally if you have been advised on a course of action based on your doctor's knowledge and experience, it is unfair to pressurise your doctor into following another course if he or she has serious medical reservations about it. And remember that your doctor's sole aim is to help you bring your baby into the world with the minimum risk to either you or your baby.

Caesarean sections can be categorised into two groups — elective and emergency. Those planned during the antenatal period are known as elective caesarean sections. Emergency caesarean sections are performed if some life-threatening complication occurs either during the pregnancy or during labour which means that it is vital the baby is delivered as quickly as possible. If the complication is severe haemorrhage, for example, or prolapse of the umbilical cord, the emergency will be considered acute; in this situation time is an absolutely critical factor and the operation will be carried out under general anaesthetic as soon as possible. Unfortunately, the emphasis on speed may also mean that there is little time for explanations. On the other hand, if your labour is not progressing for some reason, or the baby is just beginning to show signs of distress, the time factor is slightly less crucial and the doctor has longer to prepare his team and you for the operation.

It had been explained to me that as I had a rather small pelvis and a rather large baby, a caesarean section might be necessary, but I was allowed a trial labour as I desperately wanted a normal birth. My progress was explained to me by the staff and at the end of 15 hours they advised the operation due to exhaustion on my part. They gave me a little time just in case, and even at the last minute, when I had been prepared for the operation, examined me to make sure that a normal birth was not possible. As I had only dilated 5 cm it was impossible. My son was born under general anaesthetic a little while later. I was just thrilled when I held him in my arms.

Sandra

ELECTIVE CAESAREAN SECTION

There are certain complications of pregnancy, detectable during the antenatal period, which make normal vaginal delivery impossible or highly risky.

Placenta Praevia
This is when the placenta lies in front (praevia) of the baby and is attached to the lower part of the uterus. All women who have been diagnosed as having placenta praevia are delivered by caesarean section, wherever possible, before they go into spontaneous labour.

Physiologically speaking the uterus is composed of two separate parts or segments. The upper segment is predominantly made up of muscle and is responsible for the contractions which push the baby out during labour. Once the baby has been born and the placenta expelled, the upper segment continues to contract and this prevents any bleeding from the site where the placenta had been attached to the uterine wall.

The lower segment and cervix are composed of fibrous tissue with very little muscle. Towards the end of pregnancy and during labour this lower segment stretches.

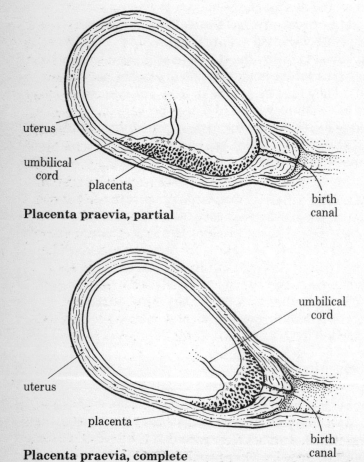

uterus

umbilical cord

placenta

birth canal

Placenta praevia, partial

uterus

umbilical cord

placenta

birth canal

Placenta praevia, complete

Normally the placenta is attached only to the upper segment, but occasionally it implants on the lower segment, either partially or entirely blocking the birth canal. The risk is that as the lower segment stretches in the last ten weeks of pregnancy, the placenta may be pulled away from the wall of the uterus, causing bleeding. The blood comes from the mother's circulation, not from the baby's, but should the loss be severe a caesarean section will be necessary to save the mother's life. If the blood loss is not too great, the mother may be given a blood transfusion to compensate for the loss and the pregnancy allowed to continue until 36 to 38 weeks, when an elective caesarean section can be performed with little risk of the baby developing breathing problems due to immature lungs.

The longer the pregnancy is allowed to continue, however, the greater is the chance that labour will start spontaneously, which would be dangerous for both mother and baby. For this reason some obstetricians recommend amniocentesis after 35 weeks of pregnancy. The sample of amniotic fluid obtained in this test enables the doctor to assess accurately the maturity of the baby's lungs. Once the doctor is confident that the baby's respiratory system is sufficiently well developed for her to breathe on her own, he can deliver the baby by elective caesarean section.

If you experience any bleeding late in pregnancy, one of the checks that will be made is for placenta praevia. The condition can be detected by ultrasound and if the scan confirms this diagnosis you will be advised to rest or stay in bed for the rest of your pregnancy. Most obstetricians prefer you to be admitted to hospital, in case any further, more serious, bleeding occurs, until the baby can be delivered by caesarean section.

Malpresentation
The most common position for a baby to lie in is with her head down (cephalic presentation), her chin tucked in and her legs flexed, with her feet crossed — the perfect position for a vaginal delivery. Occasionally, however, the baby

may lie across the uterus (**transverse lie**), especially if there is some abnormality in the shape of the uterus. If the baby is still in this position when labour starts, there is no possibility of a vaginal delivery. As a transverse lie also carries the risk that the umbilical cord might prolapse when the membranes rupture (be squeezed down out of the womb, cutting off or diminishing the blood supply to the baby), which could be fatal for the baby, an elective caesarean is usually performed for this condition shortly before the expected date of delivery.

Alternatively a baby may be lying in a **breech presentation**, meaning she is lying not with her head down, but the other way up, with her bottom presenting, or, more rarely, her feet. Babies may change their position in the womb often until finally settling into one position ready for birth. At 30 weeks of pregnancy about 25 per cent of babies are in a breech presentation, but by full term (37 to 41 weeks) only about 3 per cent are still in a

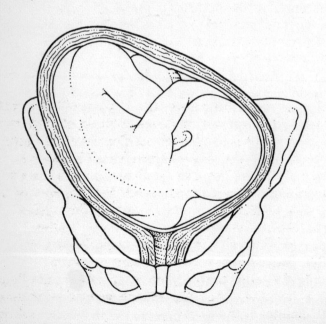

Transverse lie

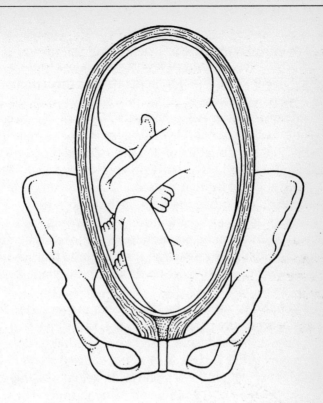

Breech presentation

breech position. In other words the majority of babies turn themselves the right way up before 36 weeks of pregnancy.

So if your baby is in a breech position before 36 weeks, do not despair — she may well turn herself round to a cephalic head-first presentation. Some obstetricians try turning the baby manually to a head-first presentation if she is still breech after 36 weeks — a procedure called external cephalic version. This is usually a painless manoeuvre, although it should only be performed by someone trained to do it. Success is by no means guaranteed — often the baby is uncooperative and will not turn, or she turns, only to flip back to her original position at a later date.

As has already been mentioned, obstetricians do not

always agree on the best method of delivering a breech baby. Some doctors will deliver all breech babies by caesarean section, in view of the two main risks inherent in breech presentation: the first being that as the baby's head, which is the biggest part of his body, is born last it may become stuck in the pelvis after the body has been delivered; and the second being the increased chance that the umbilical cord might slip down (prolapse) and become compressed as the baby's body descends, cutting off the baby's life support system too soon. Other obstetricians consider that, providing there are no other contraindications, a vaginal delivery of a breech baby can be as safe as in cephalic presentations. This is particularly so if epidural anaesthesia is used; as the urge to push is suppressed, this allows more control in the second stage of labour.

If your baby is found to be in a breech presentation in the latter part of the pregnancy, your obstetrician will conduct a number of tests to ascertain whether or not there are any other factors that would suggest that a vaginal delivery might be too risky. He will assess the size and exact position of the baby, either by palpation of your abdomen (feeling the surface of your tummy), by an ultrasound scan, by X-ray or by a combination of these procedures. (Don't worry, an X-ray at this stage of your pregnancy is not harmful to the baby as it is in the early months.) In addition he will arrange an X-ray of your pelvis to check the size and shape of the birth canal. If your pelvis is small or misshapen, or the baby is thought to be very large, he will most probably recommend an elective caesarean.

On my last visit to the antenatal clinic the doctor decided to give me an internal examination because I was so close to my due date. He announced he couldn't find the head! I was sent the next day to the hospital for an X-ray which confirmed the doctor's suspicions — James was breech and in a right pickle inside me! After studying the X-ray more it was decided I could not give birth vaginally as my pelvis looked small and considering the position he was in. Two days later, James was born by caesarean section with an epidural, which I found marvellous.

Sharan

If you have already had a baby with an easy vaginal delivery, the doctor may just assume that your pelvis is adequate and let you go ahead and try for a normal delivery. However, should any other complications of pregnancy, such as high blood pressure, have already been diagnosed, most obstetricians will recommend that you have an elective caesarean without doing any further investigations, on the grounds that the combined risk to the baby is such that an elective caesarean is by far the safer option.

Uterine Scars

If you have ever had to have surgery on your uterus, this will have left a scar. Scar tissue is much weaker than normal uterine muscle and this creates the risk that it might rupture during labour. The most common reason for operations to the uterus are caesarean section, removal of fibroids (myomectomy) and termination of a pregnancy by hysterotomy (an incision in the abdomen). If you have undergone any of these operations you should discuss the implications of your particular case with your doctor.

Usually the incision for a caesarean section is in the lower segment of the uterus, from side to side (transverse). Occasionally, however, it is necessary to make a vertical incision in the upper segment, called a classical caesarean section. (This may be done, for instance, if the baby is in transverse lie.) The classical vertical scar is considered to be weaker and more prone to rupture, so if you have had such a caesarean section previously, an elective caesarean will usually be recommended for your next birth. (Although there are exceptions to this, see Chapter 10.)

The lower-segment scar is much stronger and very

rarely ruptures. Most obstetricians would not consider one previous lower-segment caesarean section an indication for elective caesarean delivery (unless the indications for the original operation were still present, of course), but two or more previous caesarean deliveries will usually be considered too high a risk to allow labour (see Chapter 10).

A hysterotomy scar is similar to the classical caesarean scar and so an elective caesarean delivery will usually be recommended. With the removal of fibroids, if the uterine cavity has been entered, the scar is considered to be prone to rupture, but if the cavity has not been entered the doctor may suggest a trial of labour (trying a vaginal delivery to begin with, see p. 21).

Other Gynaecological Operations
If you have ever had an operation on the cervix, say a cone biopsy after an abnormal cervical smear test, it does not mean that a caesarean delivery is required. There is a risk though that any scarring may prevent the cervix from dilating normally during labour, in which case an emergency caesarean may be necessary.

If you have ever had to have a repair operation for vaginal prolapse or vaginal fistula (a hole between the vagina and bladder or rectum), then an elective caesarean delivery will normally be recommended to prevent damage to the repair.

Diseases in the Mother
If you suffer from diabetes, thyroid disease or some form of heart disease, it is possible that you will require a caesarean delivery and your doctor will advise you on whether this would be the safest course of action for you and the baby. For instance, with some heart complaints the stress of labour may be too great a risk for you, or if you suffer from diabetes there is the risk of the baby growing too large (macrosomia), meaning that it would be safer for the baby to be delivered early by caesarean section. The reduction in the risks associated with caesarean deliveries, combined with the new technology

for caring for small or premature babies, means that more and more babies who might be at risk in this way are being delivered early by caesarean section.

Vaginal Infections

Any infection that is present in the birth passage may be transferred to the baby during birth. Most vaginal infections, such as thrush (candidiasis) and TV (*Trichomonas vaginalis*), pose little threat to the baby, even if untreated.

Herpes virus, however, if transferred to the baby, can cause brain damage and even death. If you suffer from genital herpes, then you should make a careful record of the number of attacks you experience during your pregnancy, how quickly they flare up, and how long they last. After 36 weeks of pregnancy your obstetrician will arrange for tests to see if an active herpes infection is present. If the tests are positive, he will recommend that your baby be delivered by elective caesarean section as this avoids the passage of the baby through the infected birth canal.

One of the main problems with genital herpes is that although the herpes sores are easily recognised if they affect the external genitalia, if they affect only the internal organs — the cervix and vagina — there may be no obvious symptoms to raise the alarm. And, there is always the chance that an attack could occur after any test to detect the infection had been carried out. Given the severity of the damage should the baby become infected, some obstetricians prefer to deliver all babies of mothers suffering from this disease by elective caesarean.

I had suffered from herpes for about four years before I became pregnant and had learnt to live with it quite successfully. However I was very worried about the risk of transferring the disease to my baby during the birth, especially as I knew from experience that my attacks could flare up very quickly and were very often a response to fatigue. After discussing it thoroughly with my consultant we decided together that the risks were too great and opted for an elective caesarean section. I was very relieved and as it turned out I had my baby by caesarean under epidural anaesthesia with my partner by my side and it was a wonderful experience.

Lizzie

Pelvic Tumours

Occasionally routine antenatal examinations will discover the presence of an ovarian cyst or a uterine fibroid lying in the pelvis which would prevent the baby's head from descending into the birth canal. If this happens, an elective caesarean will be recommended.

Cephalopelvic Disproportion (CPD)

This is when the baby's head is too large to fit through the mother's pelvis. It is quite unusual for CPD to be given as an indication for an elective caesarean in a first pregnancy, as such disproportion is only usually diagnosed after labour has started and failed to progress. However if CPD has been accurately diagnosed in your first pregnancy an elective caesarean section would be necessary in subsequent births.

EMERGENCY CAESAREAN SECTION

Emergency Caesarean before Labour

During that antenatal period there are a number of conditions that may arise which pose a threat to the well-being of the baby or the mother, or both. One of the most common of these is high blood pressure (hypertension), which in turn may be a sign of another complication, pre-eclamptic toxaemia (PET). Your blood pressure is a fairly revealing indicator of your health during pregnancy and it will be carefully monitored at antenatal check-ups.

Why PET should occur is still not fully known. About 10 per cent of first-time mothers develop PET with varying degrees of severity, usually in the last three months of pregnancy. PET is much less likely to occur in second or subsequent pregnancies. One of the most obvious symptoms is swelling round the face, hands and ankles (again this is something that will be carefully checked at antenatal visits), but your blood pressure will also be raised and protein will appear in your urine.

In some instances it is possible to control PET with rest and drugs to lower the blood pressure. Should it develop into true eclampsia the risks to you and your baby are considerable and the baby will need to be delivered quickly. If your blood pressure can be controlled and labour can be easily induced, a vaginal delivery is possible. Otherwise the baby will have to be delivered by caesarean section.

If any of these threatening conditions are encountered, the obstetrician will not only monitor carefully the state of the mother, but will also undertake various assessments of the state of health of the baby (fetal surveillance tests). The types of test employed vary from hospital to hospital. You may, for instance, be asked to give blood and urine samples at regular intervals so that serial measurements of the hormones present can be made. Alternatively you might be given a number of ultrasound scans, so that the growth and activity of the fetus can be assessed regularly.

But the test you are most likely to encounter in these circumstances is the non-stress test (NST), otherwise known as cardiotocography (CTG) or fetal heart tracing. With this, two sensor discs are strapped to your abdomen, one to detect the baby's heart beat, the other to monitor any movement by the baby and any contractions of your uterus. The information is recorded on a paper printout as well as showing up on a small screen on the machine. The monitoring is usually carried out for 20 to 40 minutes, but may be continued longer or repeated at a later date if a clear reading is not obtained.

If this monitoring shows a drop in the baby's heart rate after a contraction of the uterus, it may mean that the baby is distressed and receiving insufficient oxygen, in which case the obstetrician will recommend that your baby be delivered as soon as possible. Whether he suggests induction of labour or emergency caesarean section depends on the degree of distress being demonstrated by the baby, the presentation of the baby, your past obstetric history and the state of your cervix — a soft, partially effaced (thin) and dilated cervix would be considered favourable for induction, but if the cervix is firm and closed this would be unfavourable.

Emergency Caesarean During Labour

From the doctor's point of view, the aims in managing your labour are to minimise any risks to the baby and at the same time to relieve the stress on you by ensuring that the labour does not continue for an unacceptable length of time. Consequently a caesarean section may become necessary during labour either because of what is called in medical terms failure of the labour to progress or because the baby is showing signs of distress.

'Failure to progress' is in many ways an unfortunate phrase. Many women who have heard this mentioned by the medical staff during their labour, and who have then had to go on and have a caesarean section delivery, focus on the word 'failure'. They, quite mistakenly, interpret it as a comment on their ability to give birth, or even on their capacity as a mother generally, and are understandably distressed. Should you be told that your labour is 'failing to progress', remember that it is purely a medical term and not a judgment of you as a woman.

The progress of your labour will be carefully monitored by the medical staff looking after you in the labour ward. There are two main indicators of progress and these will be checked at regular intervals: first, the rate at which the baby's head is descending into the pelvis; and, second, the state of your cervix. The cervix must dilate to about 10 cm (4 inches) if the baby is to pass through the cervix into the birth canal. If you imagine pulling a polo-neck sweater over your head, it will give you an idea of how the cervix has to stretch and open to let the baby's head through. The descent of the baby's head and dilatation of the cervix are plotted on your labour record or partogram, along with other relevant information.

For descriptive purposes labour can be divided into various stages, which in turn are divided into phases. The onset of labour is considered to be when regular painful contractions are accompanied by gradual thinning (effacement) and dilatation of the cervix. The first stage of labour, from the onset to full dilatation of the cervix — this is when it is 10 centimetres (4 inches), open or 'five fingers' — is divided into two phases, latent and active. The latent phase is the time from when the contractions become regular and painful to the time when the cervix is completely effaced. This phase may last up to eight hours, but it may well be over before you even go into hospital.

The active phase of labour begins when the cervix is completely effaced and ends when it is fully dilated. The rate at which the cervix dilates depends on the resistance to the descent of the baby's head and the strength of the contractions. Progress in this phase is considered 'normal' if the cervix dilates at least 1 cm (a bit less than ½ inch) per hour.

The second stage of labour begins at full dilatation of the cervix, and can also be divided into two phases. During the first phase the baby's head, pushed by the force of the contractions, descends through the cervix and down on to the muscles which form the pelvic floor. The pressure of the baby's head on these muscles causes the muscles to stretch, which triggers a reflex action. This reflex is responsible for the urge to push, which starts the second and final phase, that of the expulsion of the baby into the outside world.

Labour can fail to progress at any of these stages or phases for a variety of reasons. It may be due to cephalopelvic disproportion — the baby's head is simply too big to fit through the mother's pelvis. Alternatively the baby's head may be in the wrong position; for instance, she may be head down in the uterus but with her brow rather than the back of her head presenting — the brow is the widest part of the head and again it might simply be too large to pass through the mother's pelvis.

In some cases the contractions are just not strong enough to push the baby down through the cervix, or they may show an erratic pattern of starting and stopping. If this is the case, the obstetrician will set up a Syntocinon drip (a synthetic hormone which acts on the uterus) to try and increase the strength and effectiveness of the contractions. However if the cervical dilatation still does not reach the expected rate of 1 cm per hour, an obstruction will be suspected and a caesarean section will be performed in case further delay produces a deterioration in the baby's condition or there is the threat of the uterus rupturing.

Not only will you be carefully monitored during labour, but so will the baby. The medical staff will be looking for any sign that may indicate that the baby is distressed, meaning that the fetus might be receiving insufficient oxygen for some reason. Fetal distress is picked up by monitoring the fetal heart rate throughout the labour, using either an ultrasound transducer strapped to your abdomen (as for the non-stress test, p. 25) or an electrode clipped to the baby's scalp. Any drop in the baby's heart rate could indicate that there is a problem. Occasionally a fetal heart pattern is difficult to interpret, in which case a sample of blood is taken from the baby's scalp (this is a very safe procedure) and tested to see how much oxygen the baby is receiving.

There are degrees of fetal distress. If the distress is seen as only mild, and delivery is anticipated in a short time, labour will be allowed to continue. However, if the baby is showing signs of severe distress, the doctor will want to deliver her as quickly as possible and this will probably mean an emergency caesarean section.

In summary, a caesarean section may need to be performed for a number of reasons. Some of these are detectable during pregnancy, thus allowing for a planned caesarean delivery: others only become apparent after labour has started, requiring an emergency caesarean delivery. From the doctor's point of view, a caesarean section is done when he or she considers that the risks to the baby or mother, or to both, from continuing with labour and a vaginal delivery exceed those of caesarean delivery. With safer forms of anaesthesia this balance of risks has swung in favour of more caesarean deliveries. Indeed some doctors feel that the balance has been tipped still further in this direction by the rising expectations of what modern medicine can achieve, accompanied by an increased tendency towards litigation when these expectations are not met.

If your baby is born by caesarean section, whether it is planned or an emergency, it is important to see that it is nevertheless a birth, and as such should be a fulfilling and joyful experience. One of the keys to adopting a positive approach to this type of birth is to find a satisfactory answer to the question 'Why?' To do this you must talk to your doctor, asking him or her all the questions that will undoubtedly be in your mind, until you are given an explanation that allows you to put the operation into some perspective.

2
DECIDING FOR YOURSELF

Some hospitals suggest that a mother-to-be gives them a birth plan — a plan of how she would most like her delivery to be managed, and what she would like to happen immediately after the birth and for the first few days in hospital. This covers questions such as whether or not she would like any painkilling drugs during the delivery, and if so which ones; whether or not the father wants to be present at the birth; whether or not she would like to be handed the baby immediately after the birth; whether she wants to breastfeed or bottle-feed; how quickly she would like to leave the hospital to return home; and so on. If your baby is born by caesarean section, then obviously not all these options will be open to you, but many are and these will still need thinking through carefully. You will also have to make some choices that are specific to women whose babies are born by caesarean section, such as what type of anaesthesia to have. This means finding out as much as you can about the operation. Don't fall into the trap of thinking that, because the obstetrician is in charge of the operation to deliver your baby, you don't have any say in what is happening to you.

Many of the caesarean sections performed nowadays are elective, meaning they are planned in advance because a medical problem has been diagnosed before the mother goes into labour (see pp. 15–21). If this is your situation, you will have some time to consider the options available to you. If the caesarean section is performed unexpectedly in an emergency, it is still important to obtain information after the event to help you understand and come to terms with the operation. Find out as much as you can from the medical staff who are looking after you, from books, from other mothers, so you can make informed decisions for yourself.

It is ironic that pregnancy is not only a time for making important decisions — determining how you want things to be done for the sake of yourself, your partner and the unborn child — but is also the time when you often feel least able to make rational decisions, a time when your emotions are running away with you. Many women feel like this, so don't worry. Do try, though, to think about these questions, perhaps quietly on your own before talking them through with your partner. If you know you are going to have a caesarean section, try and find another mother whose baby was delivered this way, so she can alert you to some of the possible problems — and pleasures.

As long as you have made some effort to think things through and to find out as much as possible — from your doctor, the staff at the antenatal clinic, books, other mothers — nothing should happen that completely throws you and sends you into a state of panic. Often women who have had caesarean sections say that their biggest problem with coping was the fact of not having anticipated that this could happen to them — a caesarean section was something that only happened to other women! And this view, unfortunately, is compounded by books and pre-birth classes that just gloss over caesarean sections without ever mentioning that approximately one in nine births end this way today. So ask your questions, voice your concerns and demand some answers.

After going to antenatal classes and being told all about labour and birth, I look back now and realise that at no time was caesarean birth ever discussed in detail. If I had only known more about the operation I'm sure I wouldn't have been so shocked when it happened to me. It's not knowing or understanding what's happening to you that's so frightening.

Sally

WHICH ANAESTHETIC?

If you know in advance that your baby is to be born by caesarean section, one of the most important choices to consider is which type of anaesthetic to have — a general anaesthetic, where you will be 'asleep' for the duration of the operation, or an epidural anaesthetic.

The latter completely numbs the lower half of the body, so no pain is felt, but you remain fully conscious and alert throughout the delivery. You cannot see the actual operation in process because a screen is placed over your body at chest level. Even so some people cannot imagine being awake while a surgeon operates on them and find the whole idea very distressing. If this is you, fair enough. It's not a procedure that's right for everyone, and the only important consideration is that you are completely comfortable with what is happening to you. So don't let anyone pressurise you into having an epidural if you are hesitant about it. Remember, what is paramount is the health of your baby and your own feelings of physical and emotional well-being.

My husband and I had talked about my having an epidural anaesthetic and I knew that he was keen for this to happen so that he could be there in the operating theatre. I went along with this for a while, but finally I had to admit that I just couldn't bear to go through with it; the idea of being awake while it was happening made my toes curl up with horror! As it turned out I had the operation under general anaesthetic much to my relief, and my husband was overjoyed when he was brought our little girl to hold as soon as she was born.

Joan

My first child had been born as an emergency section under general anaesthetic and the whole thing had been really traumatic. For my second child, however, it was an epidural caesarean with my husband present throughout. It was a wonderful experience. I saw my baby son the moment he was born and we were able to cradle him in our arms just minutes afterwards.

Dee

If the operation is being performed under emergency conditions, it is very unlikely that you will be able to choose between an epidural or a general anaesthetic. An epidural anaesthetic takes about 20 to 30 minutes before it becomes effective, so if time is a vital consideration, a general anaesthetic is the only choice as it can be administered more quickly. If, on the other hand, a caesarean section is considered because the labour is not progressing satisfactorily but the situation is not one of dire emergency, an epidural anaesthetic may be offered. This is particularly likely if an epidural is already in place as part of the management of pain during labour.

What is Epidural Anaesthesia?
The sensations from the lower part of the body travel up the body to the brain in the bundle of nerve fibres that constitute the spinal cord. By administering a dose of local anaesthetic at a point in the lower back into the area between the spinal bones and the spinal cord, it is possible to numb these sensations, removing any feelings of pain in the lower half of the body while the person remains fully conscious.

For the anaesthetic to be administered, you will be asked to lie on your side and to curl up into a ball, pulling your knees up and tucking your chin in towards your chest. This is not an easy position to hold when you are nine months pregnant, but it is necessary so that the anaesthetist can locate the spaces between the spinal vertebrae — the spinal bones — in your back. Some anaesthetists prefer the mother to sit on the edge of the couch, with her feet placed on a stool and her elbows resting on a table in front of her, so she can lean forward while arching her back.

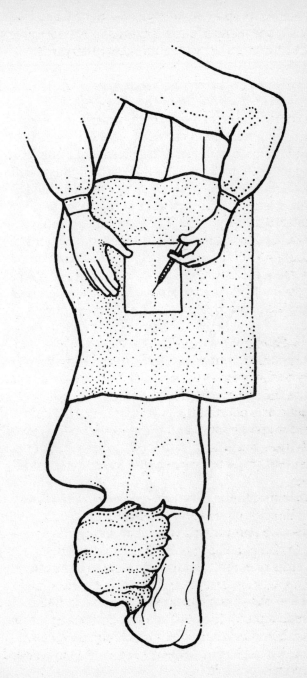

Administration of the local anaesthetic prior to the siting of the epidural

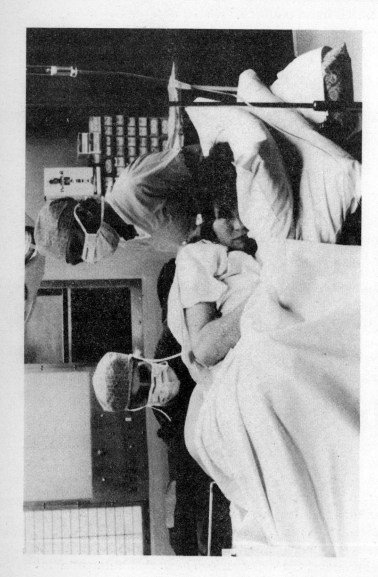

Administration of the epidural anaesthetic

Once the anaesthetist has decided where exactly he is going to administer the epidural anaesthetic, he gives a local anaesthetic to numb the skin in the lower back. This just feels like a pinprick. When this has taken effect, he then inserts a very fine needle between the bones of the spine, into the cavity between the bones and the sheath or casing of the spinal column. A very narrow plastic tube or catheter is then threaded through the needle and once this is in position the needle is removed. The anaesthetic fluid is then injected through the catheter to numb the nerve routes. Top-ups of anaesthetic fluid are given through the catheter as required.

This part of the procedure can take just a few minutes or half an hour as it is important that the anaesthetist is completely satisfied that the epidural needle is correctly positioned. The numbing effect starts shortly after the anaesthetic has been administered, starting from the feet and working upwards to about the middle of the ribcage. Once the anaesthetist is sure that you are completely numb in the lower half of your body, you are ready for the operation to begin.

If at any time during the operation you feel that you cannot cope after all, you can tell the anaesthetist; he or she will be standing by your head in the operating theatre and may decide to administer a general anaesthetic.

The Advantages

Epidural anaesthesia has some definite advantages over a general anaesthetic. It is considered to be much safer from the mother's point of view and has a minimal effect on the baby. A major consideration is that the mother is awake and alert through the whole procedure. This means she can take an active role in the birth of her child, welcoming her as soon as she appears, as with a vaginal delivery. Many women have reported how much this meant to them — the first glimpse of their baby and that unforgettable first cuddle.

Many fathers, too, hope to enjoy these first moments with their baby and a big bonus of epidural anaesthesia is that the majority of hospitals allow the father to be present in the operating theatre when this type of anaesthetic is used. This means that the couple can share what must be one of the most special events of their lives. A surprising number of men claimed that being there for the birth helped them greatly in their future relationships with their children.

From the mother's point of view, the father's presence provides her with a much-appreciated familiar hand to hold. Operating theatres are busy places and the staff may be absorbed in their specific tasks. Having someone by her side who can keep her informed as to what is happening is extremely reassuring and comforting. It also helps the progress of the operation if the mother remains calm and relaxed.

Some hospitals have a policy of leaving the epidural in place for about 24 hours so further top-up doses of anaesthetising drugs can be administered in order to manage any pain in the post-operative period. The advantage of this is that the drugs used deaden the pain while leaving the mother alert and able to hold her baby. Normally the pain experienced after the surgery is controlled with injections of pethidine, but these make the mother feel drowsy and confused and unable to take much interest in her baby. Ask your consultant what the policy is in your hospital for managing post-operative pain.

The Disadvantages

One practical problem is that not all hospitals are able to offer a woman epidural anaesthesia as it requires a skilled anaesthetist or an obstetrician specially trained in the procedure to administer and monitor it. Also those hospitals where it is available may not be able to offer it over a 24-hour span, again because of the problem of having specially trained staff on duty at all times of the day and night.

In a few cases the epidural anaesthetic fails to work, or only works down one side of the body. Should this happen, a general anaesthetic would have to be administered.

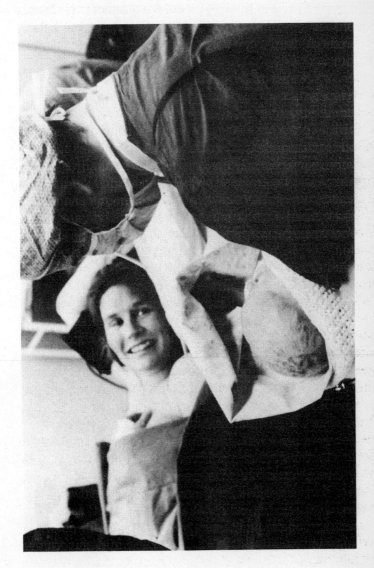

Father holding his newly delivered child following an epidural caesarean birth

Some medical conditions would indicate that it would be unwise to use this form of anaesthesia anyhow. Low blood pressure is one such example. Your blood pressure may drop dramatically with an epidural and if it is already low this could be dangerous. Equally, if you have a history of back trouble it would probably be recommended that you had a general anaesthetic instead. So the first step is to talk to your doctor at your antenatal clinic to find out what is available at your hospital and if you would qualify medically for an epidural. If it is a possibility, ask to talk to one of the anaesthetists, so you can discuss in detail the ins and outs of each type of anaesthetic.

What Happens With General Anaesthesia?

The skill in administering a general anaesthetic is to give sufficient anaesthetic to render the mother unconscious for surgery, without anaesthetising the baby too. It is crucial that the baby is delivered in a wakeful state so that she can expand her lungs and start breathing immediately. Consequently timing is all important.

Most of the preparations are completed before you are taken into the operating theatre, including having an antacid drink to neutralise the acid contents of your stomach. Once in the theatre an oxygen mask is placed over your nose and mouth; this is primarily for the baby's sake, to give a charge of oxygen in the bloodstream before the operation begins. The anaesthetising drugs are then administered through an intravenous drip and you will drift off to sleep within a couple of minutes. As soon as you are unconscious, a tube is passed down your throat into the windpipe and a combination of oxygen and anaesthetising gases are blown through it by a ventilator.

The operation moves forward with reasonable haste from this moment, because of the need to get the baby delivered before too much anaesthetic has crossed the placenta from the mother's bloodstream to the baby's bloodstream. From the time the anaesthetic takes effect to delivery of the baby is usually in the region of 10 to 20 minutes. Once the baby has been delivered the anaesthetic can then be deepened while the longer stage of removing the placenta and sewing up the many layers of the mother's abdomen is underway.

When the operation has been completed, you are taken to the recovery area until you are fully conscious and then transported up to the ward. Usually your partner can join you in the recovery room, to greet you as you come round. If all is well with the baby, she will have been handed to her father for a cuddle, so you will be able to see her in her father's arms as you open your eyes.

The Advantages

When speed is a critical factor because you or the baby are in distress, a general anaesthetic is essential as it can be administered quickly and reliably. This is why for many emergency caesarean sections there can be no choice in the matter. A general anaesthetic is also easier to administer than an epidural.

If the labour has been a long and difficult one, the thought of a general anaesthetic can come as something of a relief.

> When I was told that I would have to have a caesarean I remember being incredulous. The term fetal distress was bandied about a lot but by that time I didn't understand and didn't care. After it was decided that I would need to have the operation I relaxed a great deal — I think it was because it was all taken out of my hands. I could lie back and go to sleep and get it all over with.

> *Carol*

The mother's medical history may demand a general rather than an epidural anaesthetic. If she has low blood pressure, for instance, it would probably be safer to have a general anaesthetic as blood pressure drops less with this than with an epidural. Other medical conditions, such as multiple sclerosis or back problems, mean that a general is the only option. Occasionally some women are allergic to epidural drugs and would therefore have to have a general anaesthetic.

For some women the major advantage of a general anaesthetic is that they are unconscious and therefore completely unaware of the fact they are being operated on.

The Disadvantages

For the mother the major risk with a general anaesthetic is of regurgitating and subsequently inhaling the acidic contents of the stomach, a complication that is rare but can prove fatal. This danger is present whenever a general anaesthetic is used, but it is greater for a pregnant woman because her stomach does not empty as effectively as it does normally. However both the antacid drink taken beforehand and a number of standard safety precautions carried out as the anaesthetic is being administered minimise this risk.

For the baby the risk is that too much time will elapse between the administration of the anaesthetic and the delivery, allowing anaesthetic to travel over the placenta and enter the baby's bloodstream. As a consequence the baby is groggy on delivery and slow to start breathing, which could create further medical problems. However it should be said that the risks to both mother and baby have been considerably reduced by modern techniques, new safer drugs and more accurate monitoring.

The after-effects of a general anaesthetic can be unpleasant, although they vary considerably from woman to woman. Some women feel woozy and perhaps nauseous for a few hours after regaining consciousness and then feel fine: others feel groggy and unwell for a couple of days. The lungs tend to fill up with mucus after a general anaesthetic and coughing to clear them can be painful because of the abdominal wound. Fortunately modern anaesthetic drugs allow for very light doses to be administered, which means that the recovery time needed has been reduced.

Sometimes the baby is a little dopey for the first couple

of days, and this can bring problems with establishing breastfeeding. It is usually possible to overcome most feeding difficulties, though, with help from the midwives and a little perseverance and patience (see pp. 109–21).

Perhaps the biggest disadvantage of a general anaesthetic is that you are asleep and so miss the birth of your child. For some women this is a minor consideration compared with the safe delivery of a healthy baby. For others it causes great distress, and sometimes these mothers become depressed and have difficulty establishing emotional ties with their babies.

THE ROLE OF THE FATHER (OR FRIEND)

The question of whether or not the father is present at the birth of his child is very much one that has to be decided by the couple themselves — providing, of course, it is an option available to them in the first place. It is not always a simple decision to make. Some men may well echo Billy Connolly's feelings that 'birth is definitely not a spectator sport'. Others, on the other hand, may agree with Roger:

It didn't seem to matter about all the people there — the doctors and the nurses in their masks and gowns — I just held on to Elaine's hand. I felt terribly emotional and when they held up my son by his feet over the screen as he was born so we could see him, I couldn't help crying with joy. I was elated — and so were the staff. It was the most moving experience of my life and I wouldn't have missed it for the world.

It helps enormously if the father has had a chance to attend a few of the antenatal classes with you and has at least some idea of what to expect — and what is expected of him. If an elective caesarean section is recommended it is important he accompanies you in discussions with the consultant. Many obstetricians actively encourage the father to attend if the operation is done under epidural anaesthetic. They realise that he can provide the best emotional support for his partner, and his presence frees the staff from this task so they can concentrate on the medical requirements of the operation.

If the father does wish to be in the operating theatre, he will have to wear a gown, a paper hat and a mask, the same as the other staff. In some hospitals he may be allowed to stay with you while the epidural is administered: in others he will be asked to leave and then be reunited with you in the theatre. These sorts of decisions vary from hospital to hospital, even from anaesthetist to anaesthetist, so it is worth asking well in advance what the hospital policy is and putting in your requests to the medical staff caring for you.

During the operation itself he will be asked to sit up by your head — and to stay there, concentrating on you rather than on the surgical aspects of the operation. Once the baby has been delivered and the paediatrician has completed the first checks, she will be handed to him so he can show her to you and help you cuddle her. It is surprisingly difficult to cuddle a baby while lying down with a blood pressure cuff on one arm and a drip in the other, so the father's helping hand can be of great assistance in this manoeuvre.

Some couples like the father to be able to take photographs of the birth, and again this is something to clear with your obstetrician as early as possible.

There is no doubt that, although many men find the birth one of the most rewarding and exciting times of their lives, others consider it too stressful to watch someone you love being operated on and feel that they just could not be supportive in such a situation. Certainly if they are the squeamish sort, they are better out of the way! Equally, not all women actually want their partners to witness such an event. In both cases neither party should be pressurised into doing something they would rather not. Talk it through carefully and be honest with each other about your feelings.

If the father decides he doesn't want to be there but you would like a familiar person with you, some hospitals will allow a friend or parent to accompany you. Again this depends on the individual obstetrician, so talk to him and see if it can be arranged.

If the caesarean delivery is carried out under general anaesthetic it is unlikely that the father will be allowed to be present. Most obstetricians feel that it is distressing to the father to see the woman he loves in such a condition. In some hospitals he is allowed to wait immediately outside the operating theatre and even watch through the windows in the door. Again, the baby may be brought to him as soon as the initial checks have been made, so he is the first to greet the baby. If this is what you would like to happen, tell your doctor.

It is a good idea if the father can take a photograph of the newborn at this time, or even better ask if it is possible for one of the staff to take a polaroid photograph of the moment of birth. Not all hospitals will agree to this, although some have polaroid cameras available especially for this purpose. It can make a great deal of difference to how the mother feels about the birth and her new baby, so it is worth asking. Often women whose babies have been delivered under general anaesthetic say that they found it difficult to accept the baby as theirs because they had not been able to see her born; a photograph of the birth itself or of the newborn in her father's arms may help her overcome these feelings.

BOTTLE OR BREAST?

An important decision that any mother has to make is whether to bottle-feed or breastfeed her baby. This is a decision that only you can make, but it might help to clarify a few points if you talk to other mothers about how they fed their babies and also discuss it with your health visitor or midwife. Some of the pros and cons of both methods of feeding are examined in Chapter 7, and this might help you make up your mind if you are unsure which to choose.

The most important point is that having a caesarean

section delivery in no way prevents you from breastfeeding your baby should you wish to do so. The midwives in the postnatal ward will be able to show you ways of holding the baby that do not put pressure on your wound, and your milk will be unaffected by the operation.

HOW LONG SHOULD YOU STAY IN HOSPITAL?

Most hospitals recommend that you stay in hospital for six to ten days after the birth. Obviously much will depend on how quickly you recover from the operation and, as already mentioned, this varies considerably from woman to woman. Some mothers are bright and perky and looking after their babies within a day or a couple of days; others feel groggy and uncomfortable for longer, so would be better staying in hospital, with the back-up of the nursing staff, for as long as possible.

The important point to bear in mind when thinking about this question is that you have not only given birth but you have also undergone major abdominal surgery. This means that it will take longer for you to recover than the woman in the next bed who has had a straightforward vaginal delivery. (Although if she has had an episiotomy she may be feeling even more uncomfortable than you are!) You will have to rely more on the staff to help you with caring for your baby and generally encouraging you back on your feet. But it does not mean you have to think of yourself as an invalid — quite the opposite, a positive attitude is one of the major factors influencing the speed of recovery. But you must also be fair to yourself — and your partner and the baby.

I decided to think positive. I made a conscious effort not to think of it as just surgery, but as BIRTH. By 20 hours after my caesarean (under epidural anaesthetic) I had had a shower, washed my hair and sat in a chair to feed my baby.

Christine

Some women who have had caesarean sections do say that they felt it took them a little longer to establish a successful breastfeeding routine than other women who had had vaginal deliveries. The knowledge and support of the midwives can be especially valuable if difficulties do arise and this may be another reason not to rush home too quickly.

Much will depend, too, on what help you are able to arrange for when you do go home. This is one of the things that is worth organising well in advance. If you can ask friends and/or relatives to come in to do the day-to-day chores — shopping, cooking and cleaning — then you will obviously be in a better position for leaving the hospital early, providing your medical condition and the baby's health allow it. Take whatever help is offered at this time, so you can reserve all your energies for recovering from the operation and getting to know your new baby. If you do not have any family near at hand who can help you, it might be worth asking at your local social services department if it would be possible to arrange for a home help to come in for a few hours a day in the first week. (It is a legal obligation of the social services department to provide a home help for a newly-delivered mother if required, so do not be put off if your enquiries aren't answered satisfactorily.)

3
PLANNING AHEAD

One advantage of an elective caesarean section is that you know the exact date your baby will be born and can organise everything in advance. The other side of that coin is that you will need to be more organised than if you were having a vaginal delivery. Your stay in hospital will be longer, for instance, varying from six to ten days depending on how you and your baby progress. This means you will have to make fail-proof arrangements to cover your absence if you have other children to care for.

You will also be more physically debilitated than with a vaginal birth. A caesarean section is not just birth, it is also major abdominal surgery, and as with any operation it will take time to recover from the effects. Although you should be up and around quite quickly after the delivery, it will be some time — maybe months — before you feel fully back to normal. And it is essential that you are able to rest and recuperate as much as possible in the first few weeks if your recovery is to be rapid and complete.

Given the demands of a new baby and, if this is your first child, the trials of adapting to a new role as a mother, it is not going to be possible to convalesce in the true sense of the word, but you can certainly try and make sure that the bulk of your energy reserves are kept for you, your baby and, not forgetting, your partner. This means delegating as many of the daily domestic chores — cooking, cleaning, shopping, doing the washing — as possible and then forgetting about them. If friends and relatives offer to help with such tasks, accept gratefully. If your partner is willing and useful around the house, perhaps he can take two weeks leave after the birth to give you a hand. This has the added bonus of giving him the chance to share in the enjoyment of this new little person who has turned his world upside down.

If you do not have people around who can help in this way, it would be well worth seeing if you can afford to hire some help for a week or two — someone to come and clean and cook a meal every morning, say. Although it is not a service that is much-publicised, you do in fact have a right to the assistance of a home help supplied by the local social services department for a period of 10 days following a caesarean delivery. Some local departments insist on doing a means test to assess whether or not you should make a financial contribution for this service, but even so it may well be a more affordable way of getting some domestic support at this crucial time. Ask your health visitor for details or enquire at your local social services office.

ORGANISING THE HOME

Any plans you have been hatching for major home improvements, or even for minor decorating schemes, should be carried out now; DIY will be the last thing you will feel like doing after the baby's arrival. Similarly with spring cleaning, cupboard building and all the other activities that seem to be triggered off by the nest-building instinct experienced by most expectant parents — do them now, because it will be too much for you after the event.

It will pay, too, to think ahead about stocking up supplies of basic foods and household items so you do not have to worry when you return from hospital. If you have a freezer, prepare as many complete meals in advance as you can, so you and the family can just live out of the freezer for a week or so. Also stock up on tinned and dried goods — tins of beans, spaghetti, rice, etc., for quick easy snacks and meals. Include in the stocking-up campaign basic items such as toilet rolls, washing powders, and so on.

Now is also the time to check that all labour-saving

devices, such as the washing machine, are in functioning order. A broken washing machine could mean a broken spirit, if it is a matter of disappearing under a mountain of dirty nappies because the repair man cannot come for a week. If you can afford it, you might decide to invest in some new equipment. For instance, a number of mothers put a microwave high on their list of helpful pieces of equipment. As one mother who bottle-fed her baby pointed out:

> I can warm her bottle in 50 seconds in the microwave, compared with 10 minutes it used to take when I had to warm the milk by standing the bottle in a basin of hot water. If my baby is hungry and crying for her feed, especially in the night, saving those few minutes can do a lot for the baby's temper and my nerves!

BUYING BABY EQUIPMENT

It is unlikely that you will feel like embarking on major shopping expeditions towards the end of your pregnancy, and you will certainly not be physically up to it for quite a while after a caesarean section. With this in mind, try and do any shopping for basic requirements well in advance, while you still have the energy and enthusiasm to shop around for price and quality.

If you do not want to buy too much equipment at this stage, you can at least do the research now to check out the various options offered by different shops. There is a bewildering amount of baby equipment available these days — much of which you will not need! Once you have looked round and selected what you think is most suitable for your needs, you can always make a list of the items together with the shop supplying them. Your partner can then go and purchase what items you require before you return from the hospital.

Another possibility is buying secondhand equipment. Check the advertisements in the local paper or on the board at the child health clinic, or contact a local National

Childbirth Trust (NCT) group to see if mothers want to sell any equipment they are no longer using. But be sure to watch for any safety hazards on secondhand stuff.

Essentials

The first priority is to decide on a bed for your baby. This can be a carrycot, a Moses basket, a crib, a cradle or a full-size cot — anything, in fact, that is warm, draught-proof and safe. Then you will need bedding, either sheets and blankets (and quite a few sheets, as they will need frequent washing) or a washable baby duvet and covers. You will not need a pillow until the baby is one year old or more, as very young babies can easily suffocate with a pillow.

Another major item of equipment is the pram. Again the choice today is huge, from the traditional coach-built pram (not a very practical idea if you live in an upstairs flat) to the carrycot on wheels and the reclining buggy. The carrycot on wheels is one of the most popular combinations because the carrycot can double up as a bed and be used for travelling in the car. If you do intend to use a carrycot in the car, be sure to fit the proper restraints. Once the baby is sitting up, the wheels part of the combination can be converted into a pushchair. If you prefer the idea of the reclining buggy or pushchair make sure that it will allow the baby to lie out flat; it is harmful to a young baby's back muscles to be forced into a sitting position for any length of time before they are sufficiently developed to do so.

When choosing a pram, watch for a few fundamental points.

- It should have a sturdy framework.
- The brakes must be efficient.
- The handle should be at the right height for you, not too low or you will have to bend over to push it and this could give you back pain.
- If it is the folding variety, it should be lightweight and fold simply into a compact shape that is easy to handle.

For transport in a car, you can put the baby in the carrycot on the back seat provided the carrycot is restrained by the proper fitted straps. Also ensure that if a carrycot is to be used for this purpose it has a robust rigid frame — many carrycots seem to be made of little more than cardboard covered in material and these will just buckle if the carrycot is thrown against the restraining straps in an accident.

Alternatively you could buy or hire one of the new car seats that are available. These are suitable for very young babies and are held in place by the existing seat belt so have the advantage of not requiring any special straps to be fitted. Research has shown such seats to be one of the safest ways for a baby to travel in a car. They have the added bonus of being portable, so can be used equally effectively in the house or even popped into a supermarket trolley when you do the shopping.

A selection of baby clothes to see you through the first month is also essential. Basic requirements would include six stretch all-in-one suits (these are good for wearing in the day or for sleeping in at night), six vests, two cardigans, a hat and a shawl. If your baby is due in the winter months, you will need a woolly suit with leggings and some mittens. Bear in mind, though, that several layers of garments are better at keeping in warmth than one heavy layer.

If you are intending to use terry nappies, the advice is that you will need at least two dozen to avoid running out! And do not forget all the other things you need for terry nappies — nappy pins, plastic pants, nappy liners, sterilising powder and a bucket with a lid for soaking. Alternatively buy two large boxes of the smaller sizes of disposable nappies.

You will be spending a lot of time changing nappies once your baby has arrived, so get a plastic changing mat and find a place to put it which is at the right height for you. Bending over to change a nappy on the floor can be very painful when you have an incision, not to mention a strain on your already overworked back. Keeping your baby clean will also require you to have a baby bath at hand (a washing-up bowl will suffice), as well as towels and plenty of cotton wool, baby wipes, baby lotion, baby cream and baby soap. Again be sure it is all at a suitable height for you, bearing in mind the restrictions imposed by the wound.

Some mothers know in advance that they would prefer to bottle-feed rather than breastfeed their babies. If this is you, you will need to equip yourself with at least four bottles with teats, a steriliser and the necessary sterilising liquids or tablets, a bottle brush for scrubbing out the bottles and some baby milk powder. There are a number of different brands of baby milk currently available and your midwife or health visitor should be able to advise you on this and all the other equipment you require for bottle-feeding.

PREPARING TO GO INTO HOSPITAL

You can make your stay in hospital much more comfortable by thinking through what you might need while you are there, bearing in mind you will be in hospital for between six and ten days, compared with the two or three days most mothers stay after a vaginal delivery. There are lots of little things that can help you feel more comfortable and lift your spirits in the time just after the birth, and all those listed below have been suggested by women who have themselves had caesarean section deliveries.

You will not need to take everything in with you on day one, but pack a suitcase to cover all your basic requirements and have it ready at hand a couple of weeks before you are due to go into the hospital. Leave clear instructions as to where your partner or a friend can find clean nightdresses, towels, or anything else that you think you might need during your stay in hospital.

Basic Requirements

- **Nightdresses**. Take a couple of old ones, because for the first day or two you will probably lose a fair amount of blood, and two pretty ones to brighten up your spirits and boost your self-confidence once you are up and about again. Nightdresses and dressing-gowns will be the full extent of your wardrobe for a week or so, so you might as well wear ones that make you feel good. If you plan to breastfeed, choose nightdresses that have concealed openings or buttons down the front to facilitate the exercise.
- **Dressing-gown**. Don't take your winter-wonder thermal one. Postnatal wards are fairly tropical places, for the sake of the newborn babies, so something like a lightweight cotton one is best. However, be sure that it is comfortable and easy to wear and will not leave you feeling unnervingly exposed when the ward fills up with everyone's visitors.
- **Slippers**. Make sure they are ones you can slip on and off your feet easily (you won't be able to bend down to ease on a shoe for a while) and have non-slip soles.
- **Knickers**. Forget the sexy little lace numbers and opt for a pair of voluminous 'granny' knickers, i.e. cotton with a high waist. They might look a bit odd but they are so much more comfortable. You will probably find that your usual underwear will rub on your wound. Some bikini knickers are cut low enough to avoid catching the scar, but most mothers have said that high-waisted loose or stretch knickers are by far the most comfortable for the first week at least.
- **Sanitary towels**. In common with all women who have given birth, you will have quite a heavy vaginal flow for the first few days, and some blood loss (lochia) for the next two to four weeks, so STs are essential. Some hospitals provide these, some will offer them for the first day or two and then ask you to provide your own, while others do not provide them at all. So be

prepared. Take a packet of the stick-on variety with you for heavy flow; these are best as a sanitary belt will rub on the area of the wound and aggravate it.

- **Nursing Bras**. Take in at least two bras, preferably ones with cotton rather than elastic straps. If this is your first baby you will probably be amazed at just how huge your breasts become as they fill up with milk, and good support is essential for your comfort. Buy nursing bras from a shop that has staff trained at fitting them, as a good fit is crucial. Remember too that you will have only one hand to undo and do up the bra, so try the various types available to see which you find the simplest to manage. Also take in nursing pads as not all hospitals supply these. If you do not want to buy the prepacked ones, just cut up squares from nappy roll or Gamgi tissue. Don't use the ones with a plastic backing as this stops air getting to the nipple and can cause soreness and even infection.

- **Toiletries**. Your usual going-away collection of toothbrush, toothpaste, etc., your make-up and a box of tissues, not forgetting shampoo — if you are in a week or more you will be longing to wash your hair by about day five. Most hospitals don't allow you to have a full bath until the stitches have been removed, but you will be allowed to shower or wash kneeling in a bath after the third day. It will give your morale a real boost if you can wash your hair and put your make-up on again.

- **Towels**. Take two in with you. Your partner can always replenish your supplies as required from home.

Extras

- **Books and magazines**. Don't think that a few days 'rest' in hospital will provide the perfect moment for starting *War and Peace* or some other great tome. Not only do postnatal wards not provide a very studious atmosphere, but you will undoubtedly find your hands full meeting the demands of your new baby. Don't be surprised either to discover that your ability to concentrate is somewhat diminished in the first few weeks (some mothers complain that this is something that can last for years after giving birth rather than weeks!), so keep your reading material fairly light-hearted, or relevant — say a book on 'How to bring up baby'.

A friend of mine had told me how she had read hundreds of books about pregnancy and birth and felt she really did know everything there was to know. But she said she hadn't bothered to read about the time after the birth; she had thought that once she had got over the birth it was all down hill and mother instinct. She was shocked to find herself completely at sea for the first few days and wished she had read all the chapters headed 'You and your new baby'! I remembered her warning when I went to have Kim and was very glad I had taken a couple of baby books in with me, especially as I had a lot of difficulties breastfeeding and found reading the books a useful back-up to the advice the nurses gave me.

Geraldine

- **Coins** for the telephone.
- **Writing paper**, envelopes, pens, your address book and stamps.

Other Tips on Extras to Have at the Ready

- A large packet of **table salt**, the larger the better. If you add salt to your bathwater it helps to ease the wound and assists the healing process. Occasionally hospitals supply salt in the bathrooms, but often you will find that it has all been used before you get to it or that the hospital doesn't supply it anyway, so it is best to have your own supplies.
- **Cream for sore nipples**. Some women find that

their nipples get very sore for the first few days of breastfeeding. Camomile cream, for instance, can be very helpful at easing soreness and preventing cracking. Again some hospitals have their own lotions and potions for this, but it helps to be prepared. If nipples do get sore it may well be a sign that the baby is not positioned correctly on the breast (pp. 113–19).

- **Medication to help combat wind pain**. Not all mothers who have had a caesarean delivery suffer from this but many women do complain of wind pain after the operation, some even claiming that the discomfort from wind is greater than that from the wound. There are things you can do to combat this problem (see Chapter 6), but it is also an idea to have at the ready some tried and tested natural remedies. Peppermint in warm water, arrowroot or charcoal biscuits, for instance, all help with the discomfort caused by wind. Getting your bowels moving again after the operation is another way to help reduce the probability of wind, and increasing the fibre content of your diet can help here. Have a supply of breakfast cereal such as All-Bran or your own muesli available in case these are not included in the hospital's breakfast choices.
- Small **foam pillow** to use when breastfeeding, to keep the weight of the baby off your scar.
- The occasional **bottle of Guinness**. Recommended by some mothers not only for its iron content but also as an aid to relaxation!

Checklist of Essentials

- Nightdresses
- Dressing-gown
- Knickers
- Sanitary towels
- Nursing bras and pads
- Toiletries
- Towels

- Books
- Coins for the telephone
- Writing materials

KIT FOR COMING HOME

Just before you go into hospital prepare a bag packed with everything you and the baby will need for coming home.

For You

- **Clothes**. Loose ones, as you will still be feeling sore around the wound and have the post-pregnancy bulge (the uterus takes about six weeks to contract to its non-pregnant size).

I was dismayed to find that not only did I arrive at the hospital in a maternity dress, but I left in one too! It was the only thing I could get on that felt comfortable and didn't rub against the scar when I walked or sat down.

Katy

Don't forget to include underwear, tights and shoes, preferably flat slip-on ones as you will still find bending down an impossibility.
- A small **pillow or cushion** to hold over the wound. This will stop the seat belt rubbing and also mean you can press down to stop your bulge wobbling about with the movement of the car. Your tummy muscles will still be very slack and every bump in the road will make your tummy bounce, which pulls on the incision and can be very uncomfortable.

For Your Baby

- **Clothes**. Vest, nappy, stretch suit, cardigan, hat and shawl. If it is cold, a woolly outdoor suit would be a good idea too.

- **Carrycot** or whatever you are going to use to transport the baby.

Getting everything organised may seem a little like trying to plan a military campaign, and you are bound to forget something. One father was so keen to rush his baby home that he remembered clothes for the baby only to forget to bring any for his wife, who had to go home in her dressing gown and slippers.

4
WHAT HAPPENS DURING A CAESAREAN SECTION?

Whether your caesarean section is a planned one or performed as an emergency measure because of problems which become evident during the course of your labour, the basic procedures are essentially similar, the only difference being the speed and urgency with which they are carried out in the emergency. However all hospitals have their own policies for surgical procedures, so some of the details given below may vary slightly from hospital to hospital. If there is anything specific you wish to know, or any special requests to make, say for the father to attend an elective caesarean section birth, talk to your doctor in advance and find out what policy your particular hospital follows. Understanding what is going to happen to you, and why, takes much of the fear out of the operation, allowing you to approach the event in at least a philosophical frame of mind, if not a relaxed one.

The timing of an elective caesarean section is dictated partly by the need to ensure that the baby's respiratory (breathing) system is sufficiently mature for her to be able to breath unaided once born, which means it is better to perform the operation as near full term as possible, and partly by the medical indications for the operation. If for instance the operation has been decided on after a diagnosis of placenta praevia (where the placenta is very low down and touching, or even covering, the birth canal) it is important that you do not go into spontaneous labour as this would run the risk of the placenta breaking away from the uterine wall during contractions. If this happened you could suffer severe haemorrhaging (bleeding). With these considerations in mind the optimum time for an elective caesarean section is around the 38th week of the pregnancy.

Once a date has been decided on you are usually asked to go into hospital the afternoon before the operation (unless of course you are already there because the doctors have been monitoring your condition). If you feel very strongly about not wanting to go in the day before the operation, say because you have other small children, you can ask your consultant if it would be possible for you to come into the hospital early on the morning of the operation itself. Consultants vary in their willingness to be flexible on this point, though it should be said most consultants much prefer you to come into hospital the day before as this allows time for final medical checks to be made, documentation to be completed and for you to be starved before the anaesthetic. The 'no food and drink from 12 midnight' rule applies even if you have elected to have an epidural anaesthetic; this is just in case the need for a general anaesthetic should arise during the course of the operation.

ADMISSION

On admission the nursing staff will complete the necessary hospital documentation and prepare case notes, as with any admission. You may have been asked many of these questions before during your antenatal care, but it does offer a chance to double check. Once this is done, you will be given a wrist band with your name on it for identification purposes. A nurse will then check your temperature, pulse and blood pressure and possibly ask you to supply a sample of urine.

Some time later you will receive a visit from a member of the obstetric medical staff, often a junior doctor in training. He or she will explain again the reason for performing the operation and ask you to sign a consent form giving your formal permission for the operation to go ahead. This is known as obtaining informed consent, so be sure you are informed fully before putting your signature to it. Read it through carefully and ask any questions you want answered about the operation now. You should be perfectly happy with the explanations offered by the doctor and your consultant before signing.

One of the clauses on the standard consent form states that no guarantee is provided that any particular surgeon will perform the operation, so it is worth asking who is scheduled to carry out your caesarean section. In most instances it will be the registrar, although sometimes it is a more junior doctor under the supervision of the registrar.

This is also your chance to remind the doctor about any special requests that may have been discussed previously with the consultant. For instance, if you are having an epidural anaesthetic it may have been agreed that your partner can accompany you into the operating theatre and be present at the birth (the majority of hospitals allow this). Alternatively, if you have opted for a general anaesthetic the father might wish that the baby be brought to him as soon as he or she has been checked over by the paediatrician or you might have asked if the birth could be photographed. Remind the doctor now of these arrangements so they can be written into your notes to avoid any problems or disappointments later.

The doctor will also ask about your medical history — again most of this will be in your notes, but it ensures nothing is overlooked — and will give you a general medical examination to check that no medical conditions which might complicate anaesthesia have arisen or been missed before. He or she will listen to the baby's heartbeat and check her position to ensure that the indication for surgery is still present. For instance, if your baby was diagnosed to be in a breech presentation, there is always the chance that she has turned spontaneously to the correct position, in which case the operation would no longer be necessary. Either this doctor or the anaesthetist who will visit you later will take a blood sample so your blood can be crossmatched in case a blood transfusion should be required during the operation. (Fortunately it is rare for a blood transfusion to be needed.)

In some hospitals the doctor may also request that a fetal heart tracing be performed to check the baby's condition. This is done by means of a small ultrasound detector which is strapped to your abdomen. The baby's heartbeat is shown on a small screen and recorded on a paper printout.

Later on you will receive a visit from the anaesthetist who will check that there are no contraindications for anaesthesia and discuss with you the pros and cons of epidural and general anaesthesia (providing of course epidural anaesthesia is available at your hospital and it is an option for you in medical terms) and explain fully the procedures involved in each. If you elect to have an epidural you will be asked to sign another consent form giving your formal permission for this procedure to be carried out.

Apart from routine checks by the nurses of your pulse, blood pressure and temperature, and the baby's heart rate, you will be left in peace for the rest of the day – or as much peace as a busy hospital ward allows. In some hospitals your partner will be permitted to stay with you for most of the time — check this out in advance if possible. Otherwise equip yourself with a good book, finish your knitting, or write all those letters to pass the time. It may feel like a long wait.

You will be offered an evening meal, usually served around 6 pm, and a bedtime drink (bedtime being rather early in hospitals), but after midnight you will not be allowed food or drink — not even a sip of water — as it is crucial your stomach is empty at the time the anaesthetic is administered. In theory you should then be free to sink into slumber for your last undisturbed night, although the inevitable activity of a hospital ward and your own excitement and apprehension may well conspire to keep you awake. Ear plugs may help if you have remembered to bring them with you, while some hospitals automatically offer sleeping pills. If you think that sleeping might be a problem for you, it is probably wise to take a sleeping pill for once; you have a long day ahead of you tomorrow and a good night's rest will help you through it.

PRE-OPERATIVE PREPARATIONS

The next day will begin rather early. Hospital routine swings into action any time after 6 am, and unfortunately in your case not with a cup of tea. However the last preparations for the delivery will soon begin, so at least you will know that the moment of birth is drawing close and this will help to keep you going. First a nurse will shave your pubic hair. This will not be a full shave; rather the instruction is to remove all visible hair from the area of the incision, which will leave you with a sort of interesting 'goatee beard' effect.

You may then be given either an enema or suppositories. Not all obstetricians make this a pre-operative requirement, but some insist that your bowels are empty during the operation, both to allow as much space as possible in that area for the surgery (which is also why the bladder must be emptied and remain empty throughout the operation) and also to avoid the risk of a bowel movement during the operation. The enemas used are small ones.

While everyone else in the ward not due to have surgery that day has breakfast it may be suggested that you take a shower or a bath. Some hospitals supply specific sterilising liquid for your bath, while others are content with normal cleanliness. All make-up and nail varnish must be removed, the latter because the anaesthetist needs to be able to check the amount of oxygen you receive during anaesthesia by examining the blood vessels in the nail bed. You will be asked to remove any dentures you may have and also to take off any jewellery and give it to the nurse for safe-keeping, with the exception of your wedding ring, which will be covered with surgical tape.

Your temperature and blood pressure will be checked once again, as will the baby's heartbeat, and you will be asked to drink a white, peppermint-flavoured liquid. This is an antacid mixture to neutralise the acid contents of the stomach as a precaution against you inhaling regurgitated stomach acid into your lungs during the administration of the anaesthetic.

You will then be asked to change into a sterile hospital gown. These are usually rather short and are fastened by three or four ties down the back. It is at this moment that you can kiss all concerns with personal modesty goodbye. More often than not these gowns fail to fit even the unpregnant form; given the extra material needed to cover a full-term bump you can be fairly sure that your rump will be exposed for general ridicule! Some hospitals like you to wear a hospital cap to keep your hair out of the way too.

FATHERS

If the father or someone else is accompanying you into the theatre, they will also be asked to dress up appropriately. A nurse will supply them with a sterile gown, a cap to cover their hair, possibly covers to put over their shoes, and a mask.

By the time James had got all his kit on I could only see his eyes, or rather his specs, but it helped so much, just being able to look into his eyes and see his calm, reassuring expression.

Liz

It is always hot in operating theatres, so he shouldn't wear too many other clothes or he may be overcome with heat and faint. Then he would have to live with the fact that everyone will assume he passed out at the sight of blood!

If you are having a general anaesthetic and your partner is not allowed into the theatre, he should ask the nurse where he should wait, preferably as close to the theatre as possible. And he should emphasise that he would like the baby brought to him as soon as possible after the birth so he can enjoy the magic of that first cuddle. If at all possible it is well worth him taking along a camera — a polaroid is best — so he can take a photograph of these early moments. It will mean a great deal to you if you are subsequently able to see pictures of these precious first minutes that you are unable to share.

OFF TO THEATRE

Shortly before the time for your operation, a hospital trolley will arrive to take you down to theatre. Your world will now become populated by people who all look rather similar, as everyone will be wearing gowns, hats and masks, and this can be very unnerving as you lie on the theatre trolley like a beached whale. Operating theatres are notoriously busy places, with a surprisingly large number of people milling about, all intent on performing their particular task and paying more attention to you as a body than to you as a person. Just bear in mind that their one combined aim is to help you deliver a healthy baby and it might make them seem less alien and alarming. The theatre staff usually consist of:

- Two **obstetricians** — the registrar or consultant who will perform the operation and another doctor who will assist.
- The **anaesthetist** and his or her assistant. If you are having an epidural anaesthetic, it is the anaesthetist with whom you will have most contact during the operation. While the obstetrician is occupied delivering the baby, the anaesthetist will be standing at your head keeping an eye on your condition and telling you what stage the operation has reached so you know what is going on.

- A **scrub nurse**, who handles all the sterile instruments.
- An **assistant nurse**, referred to as a runner because she has to do just that!
- Possibly a **midwife**, if the other nurses present are not qualified in midwifery.
- A **paediatrician** who is there to check over your baby once he or she is delivered.

If the operation is being carried out in a teaching hospital, this throng may be increased still more by the presence of students.

Usually you are taken first to one of the rooms leading off the theatre itself, where you will be met by the anaesthetist and where all the last-minute preparations are done. The first of these preparations is to ensure that your bladder is completely empty. (In some hospitals this is done in the ward, before you are bought down to the theatre.) The bladder is located just in front of the uterus, which means that the surgeon has to ease it gently out of the way to gain access to the lower segment of the uterus so that he can get the baby out. Consequently it is essential that it is empty and flat throughout the operation. To do this a nurse inserts a urinary catheter (a fine tube) into your urethra (the hole you pee out of), thus allowing the urine to drain out. The catheter is usually left in place during the operation and for some time afterwards. The procedure can be uncomfortable but should not be painful. If you have learnt relaxation exercises at antenatal classes, the techniques may be useful at this time, just to stop your muscles tensing up.

I was dreading it when the nurse came to put the catheter in, but I made myself do my breathing exercises. I don't know whether they helped or not, but I certainly didn't feel any pain, just a very slight tingling sensation. It was over before I knew it.

Jennie

If you are having an epidural, the catheter may not be inserted until after the anaesthetic has been administered, in which case you will not feel anything.

The anaesthetist then sets up an intravenous (IV) line. He does this by inserting a small needle into a vein on the inside of your arm or the back of your hand to which a plastic tube connected to a bottle of sterile salt solution (saline) is attached. The intravenous line is usually placed in your left arm, so if you are left-handed ask if it can be put in the other arm; the drip is left in place for 12–24 hours after the operation and it can be very restricting if it is placed in the hand you use most. The intravenous line usually has a small tap on it, which allows fluids to be administered on one side and any drugs required, including the general anaesthetic, on the other. The arm with the intravenous line may be taped to a board to ensure that you don't make any sudden movements which might pull the needle out.

Initially the anaesthetist will run 1 litre (nearly 2 pints) of saline (or a similar solution) through the IV. This has a two-fold purpose:

- to correct any element of dehydration that might have occurred because you have not had any food or drink for a number of hours; and
- to give your circulation a boost to ensure that your blood pressure does not drop too much when the anaesthetic is administered as this would interfere with the flow of blood to the baby.

Maintaining an adequate flow of blood to the baby is one of the principal concerns during the delivery and for this reason you will be tilted on to your left side during the administration of the anaesthetic and during the operation — either the operating table itself will be tipped slightly to the left, or a bolster wedge will be placed under your right hip. This helps shift the weight of the baby away from the major blood vessels in your body to avoid them being compressed. Should these blood vessels become compressed, the return flow of blood to your heart would be restricted, which would in turn decrease the volume of blood available for pumping back around your circulation to the baby.

A blood pressure cuff will also be strapped to your right arm so that your blood pressure levels can be checked every few minutes. In some hospitals you may also be wired up to a cardiac (heart) monitor.

THE ANAESTHETIC

Procedure for a General Anaesthetic

If you are having a general anaesthetic (see pp. 40–45) all the preparations will be completed before the anaesthetic is administered in the operating theatre. This is because it is crucial that the baby is delivered speedily once the anaesthetic has been given, to ensure that as little as possible of the anaesthetising drugs pass over the placenta and into the baby's bloodstream.

An oxygen mask will be placed over your nose and mouth so you can breathe in oxygen for about five minutes before the anaesthetic is given. This is principally for the baby's sake, to boost the oxygen levels in the blood before the birth. While the mask is in place, your abdomen will be cleaned and wiped with an antiseptic liquid and your whole body covered with sterile drapes so that only the area of the incision is exposed.

The anaesthetic is then administered via the intravenous drip and you will drift off to sleep. Just before losing consciousness, you will feel a nurse press down quite firmly on your throat. This is a precaution to prevent any regurgitation of the contents of the stomach and their subsequent inhalation, a complication which is very serious and sometimes fatal. Once unconscious, you should not know any more until you wake up in the recovery room. However, about 5 per cent of women undergoing caesarean sections claim to recall events and conversations after their anaesthetic. This is due to the very low dose of anaesthetic used prior to the delivery of the baby.

As soon as you are unconscious, you will be given a muscle relaxant and a tube will be passed down your throat, through which oxygen and anaesthetising gases are blown by a respirator. Some women have reported a sore throat after the operation from the insertion of this tube. The tube remains in place until you are sufficiently awake after the operation to regain the reflex action of coughing, then it is removed.

Now everything is ready for the operation to begin.

Procedure for an Epidural Anaesthetic

An epidural anaesthetic (see pp. 34–40) is usually administered before you are actually taken into the operating theatre, in one of the rooms off to one side. You will be asked either to lie on your left side, curled up in the fetal position, or to sit on the edge of the bed, feet on a stool, and lean forward on to your elbows. The reason for adopting these rather uncomfortable positions — uncomfortable given your size — is that the anaesthetist has to inject the anaesthetising fluid into the space surrounding the nerves as they emerge from your spinal cord within your backbone, and arching the back in this way opens the spaces between the vertebrae to facilitate this.

First the anaesthetist paints your back with an antiseptic solution— this just feels cold. Then he numbs the area in the small of your back where the epidural is to be inserted, using an injection of local anaesthetic. Once this has taken effect he inserts a slightly larger needle between two vertebrae in the spine and into the epidural space around the spinal cord. The positioning of this needle is crucial; if it is not in the right place the anaesthetic will not work properly and if it penetrates too far some spinal fluid may be drawn off and you could spend the next 48 hours flat on your back with a crashing headache. Fortunately the great majority of anaesthetists who perform epidurals are both skilful and experienced, so such errors are rare. These potential risks, however, mean that the anaesthetist will take great care in ensuring that the needle is correctly positioned and this may take some time and perhaps require more than one attempt. Concentrate on your breathing and relaxation techniques while this is happening. Although you should not experience any pain while the anaesthetist is inserting the needle, he or she will need to use a degree of pressure to push it into the spine and this can be very uncomfortable. The ease with which an epidural can be administered does vary from woman to woman:

> The anaesthetist seemed to be fiddling about for hours and I found it more and more difficult to keep curled up on my side — it was so uncomfortable, and I suddenly seemed to have got a skin as tough as a rhinoceros's from the amount of pushing it seemed to take to get the wretched needle in. This was the worst bit of the whole operation for me.
>
> *Marion*

> I was almost shaking with fright by the time I was wheeled into the anaesthetics room, but the anaesthetist was so kind and gentle, and told me exactly what he was doing all the time. I hardly felt the needle go in, just a tiny twinge and that was that.
>
> *Sarah*

The anaesthetist checks the needle is in the right place by injecting air — if the flow of air doesn't meet any resistance he knows it is correctly located. He then threads a thin tube or catheter through the needle into the epidural space. It is not unusual to experience a sharp twinge of pain down one leg as he does this, but it will only be momentary and is no cause for alarm.

The needle is then removed and the catheter is strapped up your back with sticking plaster so that the injection

CAESAREAN SECTION

end is up by your shoulder and easily accessible. A small
test dose of the anaesthetising agent is administered
through the catheter and your blood pressure levels are
watched for a reaction. If all is well, a larger dose is given.
You will be asked to turn on your right side to ensure an
even spread of the drug over the spinal nerves.

The numbness starts from your toes and works
upwards. At first your feet feel surprisingly hot and tingly,
then they feel very heavy and finally go numb. The
numbness gradually works up your body to just below
your breasts. Don't worry if you suddenly find yourself
shaking and shivering, possibly quite violently. This is a
perfectly normal response and passes off in a few
moments. Your relaxation exercises might help you here.
The anaesthetist will either prick your skin with a pin or
rub ether on your skin — this will feel cold if sensation is
still present — to check that your abdomen is quite numb.

It takes about 20 minutes for the anaesthetic to work
fully. As soon as the anaesthetist is satisfied that it has
taken effect, you are wheeled into the operating theatre.
Very occasionally the epidural does not entirely remove
sensation, in which case a general anaesthetic would have
to be administered in addition to the epidural.

In the theatre an oxygen mask is placed over your nose
and mouth so you can breathe in oxygen — for the baby's
sake — while the final preparations are completed and
surgery begins. The surgeon paints your abdomen with
antiseptic solution and then covers your body with sterile
surgical drapes, leaving only the site of the incision
exposed. There is a bar attached to the operating table
above your chest and the drapes will be laid over this too
so you cannot see your abdomen and the actual surgery.
Most women are quite glad not to witness the surgery, but
for the pluckier ones it is often possible to see what is
happening reflected in the large lights over the operating
table if you want to look.

You will undoubtedly be feeling rather apprehensive by
now, lying on your back, with a blood pressure cuff on one
arm and a drip in the other, and half of your body feeling

as though you have forgotten to bring it with you. This is when the presence of your partner can mean so much, a familiar person to hold on to, to reassure and explain what is happening. If your partner is not with you, a nurse will often sit up by your head and the anaesthetist will keep you informed of progress.

If you are anxious, do tell the staff. Often a simple explanation can put your mind at rest. And in a very short while you will be able to greet your baby.

THE OPERATION

(Note: if the medical details are not what you want to know about, skip this bit.)

The first task for the surgeon is to make an incision in the skin. The most common skin incision for a caesarean section is a transverse incision, or what is known colloquially as a bikini cut. This type of incision is preferable for a number of reasons: cosmetically it is the most acceptable because it is positioned about the level of the pubic hair line, so once the hair has regrown, the scar is almost invisible; medically it is the best option because the healing is quicker than for a vertical scar; and it is a more tolerable wound in the post-operative recovery period.

However occasionally medical reasons dictate that a vertical skin incision is used. In this the incision runs from just above the pubic bone up to just below the navel. If your baby is in a transverse lie (across the womb), for instance, the surgeon may decide to do a vertical incision if he or she anticipates any difficulties, as it allows slightly more room for manoeuvre.

After making the skin incision, the surgeon cuts through the fatty tissue just below the skin and the fibrous sheath which surrounds the abdominal muscles. The muscles themselves are then split — not cut — to reveal the peritoneum (the thin membrane of tissue which covers the entire inside of the abdomen and which also envelopes all the organs in the abdomen). Once an incision is made in

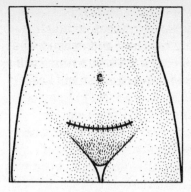 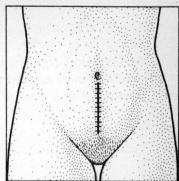

Transverse incision   **Vertical incision**

the peritoneum the uterus immediately becomes visible as
it takes up most of the space in the lower abdomen. (Your
bowel will have been pushed up out of the way as the baby
grew in the uterus.)

The peritoneum covering the front of the uterus and the
bladder is then cut and the bladder is gently eased away
from the lower segment of the uterus and pushed out of
the way. A transverse incision is made in the lower
segment of the uterus, revealing the membranes, amniotic
fluid and the baby below. (Occasionally a vertical
(classical) incision is made if a lower segment incision is
medically unsuitable. However this type of incision is
avoided whenever possible as it produces more bleeding
and is prone to rupture in a subsequent pregnancy.) The
membranes are then broken and the amniotic fluid is
removed by an electronic sucker. The surgeon inserts the
fingers of his right hand under the presenting part of the
baby to guide her out, while at the same time the assisting
doctor presses down firmly on the top of the uterus. He
does this two or three times, pushing the baby out through
the incision, not unlike toothpaste from a tube.

It is important to point out that if you are having the
operation under epidural anaesthesia, although it will have
blocked out sensations of pain, it will not have blocked out

all sensations. You will still be aware of tugging and pulling, and know when any pressure is being applied, and this can come as a shock if you have not been warned about it in advance. Most women who have had caeserean sections under epidural say that it is not a particularly unpleasant feeling, but is similar to a dentist's anaesthetic, where you do not experience any pain but you can still 'feel something' when you touch your cheek. One woman described a kind of dragging sensation when the skin incision was being made, 'as if a well-sharpened pencil was being drawn across my skin'. Another described her feelings during the operation as follows:

> I felt just like a large shopping bag, with someone rummaging around in the bottom trying to find the keys or something. It wasn't painful at all; it just felt very odd.

You will undoubtedly feel the pressure being exerted on your abdomen to push the baby out. In fact the doctor or the anaesthetist should warn you that this is about to happen as the force required to get the baby out is often considerable and it can be extremely uncomfortable to have some hefty doctor bearing down on you if you aren't expecting it.

> It was just as if a hippopotamus had sat on me — it quite took my breath away.

Lizzie

One compensation is that the part of the operation concerned with the delivery of the baby is fairly swift, only about 5 to 10 minutes. A few seconds after all the squeezing you may feel a great relief of pressure as your baby is delivered and the next thing will be your first glimpse of your baby as she is held up over the screen by her little feet, a sight that makes it all worthwhile.

After any mucus has been suctioned out from her nose

and mouth and the surgeon has clamped and cut her cord, your baby is handed to the midwife or paediatrician who will check her state of health. All babies are assessed at one minute and five minutes after the birth against what is called the Apgar score. This notes heart rate, muscle tone, breathing, skin colour and response to stimulation and rates them on a score of 0–10. A score of 8 or more means the baby is fine, between 5 and 7 may mean slight problems that need watching and a boost of oxygen via face mask, and a score of less than 5 means the baby needs resuscitation.

If the baby is deemed well and you are awake she will be wrapped up in a blanket and given to you for a cuddle. This isn't as easy as it sounds when you are lying down and have various attachments to both arms, but can be achieved with the help of your partner or a nurse.

The baby was plonked on my chest and it took a great deal of hitching and manoeuvring with the help of James before I could get her in a comfortable position, but oh, the sheer joy of holding her close, that funny little screwed up face. It was love at first sight for both of us and we burst into tears of happiness. I hardly noticed them sewing me up.

Lizzie

You will notice that the baby is covered in a greasy, cream-coloured substance; this is called vernix and it protected her skin while she was in your uterus. Often babies born by caesarean section have a better appearance than their counterparts born by vaginal delivery. In a vaginal delivery the baby's skull is moulded by its passage through the birth canal and this can produce some very odd head shapes temporarily. Caesarean section babies on the other hand, because their heads have not been squeezed on their way out into the world, have pleasantly rounded little heads.

If you are under a general anaesthetic, the baby can be taken to her father for him to hold and cuddle.

Those big blue eyes just stared straight up at me. I walked up and down, holding her close in my arms. I could hardly believe it, a whole new life, I couldn't take my eyes away from hers. A fabulous feeling.

Mike

If the caesarean section has been performed because of fetal distress, say, the baby may need immediate expert care and attention and it might not be possible for you to hold her straightaway. This can be nerve-racking and the staff should keep you fully informed about what is going on and why the baby needs special care (see pp. 88–90).

THE LAST DETAILS

Finishing off the surgery takes rather longer than the delivery itself — anything from 20 minutes to an hour. If you are awake you will probably be too busy getting to know your new baby to notice what goes on behind the screen, although you may feel some tugging as you are sewn back together again. If you have had a general anaesthetic, it is usually deepened once the baby has been delivered and the sewing up process begins.

First the surgeon removes the placenta and cleans and checks the uterus before the uterine incision is closed with sutures (stitches). As soon as the surgeon is sure all the bleeding has stopped, the various layers of the uterus and abdomen are sewn back together — a time-consuming job — and finally the skin incision is closed. How this is done depends on the surgeon, and choices range from individual sutures to skin clips or staples or a combination of these. Occasionally a single subcuticular suture (just under the surface of the skin) using either absorbable or non-absorbable material is used. If you have had a transverse incision, you will usually have a drainage tube from the wound attached to a vacuum bottle; this is to prevent an accumulation of blood within the wound that could lead to infection or breakdown of the wound. The wound is then dressed and the operation is completed.

If you have had an epidural, you may be given a top-up of anaesthetic before the catheter is removed. Alternatively some doctors leave the epidural catheter in place and use top-ups through this for post-operative pain relief rather than pethidine injections. You are now ready to be transferred to the ward, hopefully with your baby and partner by your side, to rest and recover.

With a general anaesthetic, you will be taken from the operating theatre to a recovery room so you can be carefully monitored as you gradually come round. The return of the coughing reflex is a sign that you have regained consciousness and most anaesthetists leave the endotracheal tube in place in your throat, until you cough and take it out yourself, showing that you are sufficiently recovered to breathe on your own. You will usually stay in the recovery room about half an hour before being taken up to the ward, but most hospitals will allow your partner to sit by you, with your baby if she is well (if the nursing staff do not suggest this, the father should ask). You will drift in and out of sleep during this time, but you will be able to see your baby and be reassured all is well — even if you can't remember it later!

IN AN EMERGENCY

Very occasionally a birth runs into trouble, to the degree that the situation is one of dire emergency and it is imperative that the baby is born without any further delay. Such a situation would arise, for instance, if there was a prolapse of the umbilical cord — fortunately a rare complication of labour — where the baby's umbilical cord descends first, in front of the presenting part of the baby, with the obvious risk that the cord will become compressed, cutting off the oxygen supply to the baby as it descends into the birth canal.

In an emergency such as this the medical and nursing staff go into a sort of overdrive and, unfortunately, the woman's comfort, modesty and level of anxiety may have to take second place to the need to get the baby out fast with the minimum of risk to either mother or child. This means getting the general anaesthetic administered and the operation underway at a speed which will leave little time for explanations. If this happens to you be sure to talk to the nurses and doctors after the event about exactly what happened and why, so you are clear in your mind what necessitated such abrupt action.

I just heard someone make a reference to the cord and then it was as if a fire alarm or something had gone off — all action. I was helped on to all fours and told to put my bum up in the air — very dignified, I'm sure! The doctor explained to me later that this was to take the baby's weight off the cord. Then I was rushed down endless corridors to theatre, still with my bum in the air. Needless to say it had to be visiting time! The next thing I knew I was coming round and Brian was sitting by me, holding our son. I couldn't think how it had all happened. What was the baby doing there? Then I drifted back off again. Much later the doctor came to see me and explained what had happened, that his cord had prolapsed and the need to get him out quickly. I had to laugh when a nurse described me on the trolley being wheeled at full tilt through the hospital corridors with everyone jumping out of the way — though it hadn't seemed funny at the time.

Francis

Fortunately this level of emergency does not occur very frequently. Even if a caesarean section is decided on because of a complication during labour, there is usually time for explanations of why the decision has been made and what will happen to you.

5
THE FIRST FEW HOURS

FOR YOU

Most women report that the first few hours after a
caesarean section pass in a daze, whether it be from
excitement, relief, worry if something has gone wrong, or
merely as a side-effect of the anaesthetic and the pain-
relieving drugs.

If you have had an epidural and the birth went well, you
may well feel euphoric for the first couple of hours back on
the ward. The anaesthetic is still working so you won't be
in any pain, the baby is tucked up in her crib next to your
bed for you to admire and your partner is by your side,
equally jubilant. Unfortunately, this happy state of affairs
does not last. As the epidural wears off and the feeling in
your body returns, starting with your toes and working up,
you will become aware of pain.

Control of Post-operative Pain
Everyone has a different pain threshold, and what seems
intolerably painful to one person is quite manageable for
another. However there is no escaping the fact that a
caesarean section is a major abdominal operation and any
surgery of this nature is accompanied by considerable pain
in the post-operative period. The degree of that pain for
you depends on your personal ability to cope with pain,
how well the operation went and how effective the
medication you are given for controlling it is. The most
important point is to be prepared psychologically, to
expect the wound to feel painful for the first 24 hours and

accept what painkilling drugs are suggested to help you through this time.

> The nurse had told me to let her know as soon as I got any feeling back in my toes, as this would indicate that the epidural was wearing off and she could arrange for an injection of a painkiller. Gradually I could feel my toes but I thought 'Oh, I'll wait a bit before telling the nurses — I don't want them to think I'm one of those moaning minnies.' But that was a real mistake. When I did eventually ask for some help, the pain was quite intense. The nurses seemed to be very busy with mothers coming up after delivering, so it took a while for them to arrange an injection for me, then it took a good 45 minutes for the drug to work, by which time I was really finding it quite difficult to cope.
>
> *Lizzie*

Pain medication is usually in the form of pethidine injections which should control the discomfort, so don't be afraid to ask for some help before it gets too much for you. If you don't think the painkillers are working — bearing in mind that they take about 30 minutes to be effective — tell the nursing staff, who can then consult a doctor to see if the dosage should be increased or the injections should be given more frequently.

Many mothers advise from their experience that you have regular injections of painkillers, every three or four hours, for the first day after the operation so that you can keep on top of the pain. This leaves you sufficiently relaxed to rest and enjoy your baby. One drawback of the pain medication, though, is that it can make you feel rather drowsy. Again it is better not to fight this but get as much recuperative sleep as you can. Your baby will probably want to rest peacefully in this first day of life, so why don't you?

A few hospitals follow a policy of leaving the epidural in place after the operation so that top-up injections can be given for controlling the pain when you are back on the ward. This has one considerable advantage, in that it avoids the side-effects of pethidine such as drowsiness and confusion, leaving you pain-free and alert to take an interest in your baby. The epidural is then removed after about 24 hours, when you are able to take any medication required orally.

Post-operative pain diminishes after the first 24 hours or so, and over the next couple of days you will require less and less medication to cope, until the occasional paracetamol tablet will be all you need. Keeping the pain at bay is important for two main reasons: first, it means that you are able to get up and on the move much more quickly, which will have a significant effect on the speed at which you get back to normal after the operation; and, second, you are more likely to feel up to looking after and feeding your baby. Don't worry about the drugs passing through to the baby if you are breastfeeding — very little will get into your breastmilk, certainly not enough to do any harm.

If you are coming round after having the operation performed under a general anaesthetic, you will feel rather woozy, confused and possibly nauseous for the first few hours. You may well swing in and out of sleep, speaking to your partner or one of the nurses quite normally one minute, then slipping back into sleep, only to wake again later and remember nothing of your previous conversation. The first dose of painkilling drug will be administered before you leave the recovery room and again this adds to the drowsiness and confusion, so it is best to try and just rest and sleep.

Some women recover from the after-effects of a general anaesthetic with amazing speed and feel fine after a few hours, especially as modern anaesthetics require only very light doses to be administered; other women take a little longer, feeling distinctly groggy and tired for some time. One problem with a general anaesthetic is that it often leaves you feeling very chesty as the lungs tend to fill up with mucus, and coughing to clear them can be extremely

uncomfortable as it pulls on the wound. Learning to 'huff'
rather than cough can help reduce the discomfort (see
p. 141).

One morsel of compensation is that, should you need to
have any future babies delivered by caesarean section,
more often than not the post-operative pain levels lessen
with every subsequent operation. This is because some of
the nerves cut in the first operation never regenerate.

Medical Checks

The nurses make frequent checks on your condition in
these first few hours. Your temperature, blood pressure,
urine, and vaginal discharge or lochia are monitored, and
they also check the size and shape of the uterus to see if it
is beginning to contract, although it takes about six weeks
for it to return to its non-pregnant size. The colour,
consistency (i.e. whether or not there are any clots
present) and amount of the lochia supplies an external
indication of how well the uterus is healing. Abnormalities
in the lochia may be the first sign that all is not as it
should be. Equally, if you think that the pain is not
decreasing or even that it is getting worse, do not hesitate
to tell the nursing staff as there is always the risk of
infection with any surgery. They will also check the wound
regularly to ensure that there is no sign of infection and
that it is clean and dry.

Fortunately most caesarean sections are
uncomplicated. Probably the most frequent infection
following a caesarean section is an infection of the urinary
tract due to the insertion of the catheter to drain the
bladder. If such an infection does occur it will be treated
with a course of antibiotics which are usually effective at
clearing it up quite quickly. Infections of the wound are
more rare and more difficult to get rid of, although a
course of antibiotics is usually sufficient to deal with these
infections too.

The IV drip is left in your arm for the first 12 to 24
hours, or until you are able to drink enough to maintain
your liquid levels unaided. In many hospitals the urinary

catheter is also left in place for the first few hours after the operation, but it will be removed as soon as possible (the removal of the catheter is not painful). Passing urine is another sign that the system is returning to normal and the nursing staff will encourage you to use a bedpan within 12 hours of the operation.

The presence of the drip and the catheter, combined with the wound itself, make movement in these first few hours very difficult and you will need help when you want to cuddle or feed your baby. Remember that the nursing staff are there to support you in looking after your baby, so don't be afraid to ask for assistance and don't think you will be considered a nuisance if you do so.

Emotions

You may feel surprised by your feelings towards your baby immediately after the birth. Perhaps maternal love has not come gushing forth as you expected and you now feel a genuine sense of anticlimax. If you had an emergency caesarean section and are feeling shocked by what has happened and ill from the anaesthetic, you might find it difficult to focus on the baby at all. If you had a general anaesthetic and so not witnessed the birth you may be harbouring some suspicion that this is not really your baby — she is so different from the image you have been carrying around in your mind for the last nine months. Don't panic. Many women experience such feelings, particularly if the birth has been a difficult one. (See Chapter 8 for a detailed discussion.)

Give yourself time to recover and, as you feel better, cuddle and hold the baby as often as possible so you can get to know this little stranger. Love isn't something that flows in automatically after the birth, like breastmilk. It often needs time to form and grow.

I felt really weird for about the first day after the operation. I kept waking up and seeing this little bundle lying in the perspex cot by my bed but I didn't feel anything. It seemed as though I had waited and worked for this moment and now it was all nothing. I felt quite empty. The next day I cuddled him as often as I could, but I'd still got this empty feeling. David was ecstatic about his son and it was impossible for me to explain how I felt. It wasn't really until we came home that I began to feel love for him. He's three months old now and I adore him. I realise now that it just took us a while to get to know each other, but I was scared by my lack of feeling to start with.

Penny

On the other hand it may have been love at first sight and, despite the discomfort and immobility, you feel over the moon with happiness.

She had a round little red face, all screwed up with a button nose and a rather blotchy skin. I'm sure everyone who came to see her thought what a funny little thing, but to me she was the most beautiful baby in the world. I was completely besotted with her and just wanted to hold her all the time, even though it was hard to get comfortable with her in my arms.

Jennifer

It can be immensely reassuring to have your partner close by in these first few hours, if the hospital allow it. You may well be feeling overwhelmed, emotionally and physically, by the experience of birth and the after-effects of the operation, and a familiar hand to hang on to is a great comfort. He can also be a positive practical help, a role he might relish after being rather on the sidelines during the operation. Postnatal wards are surprisingly busy places and it is invaluable to have someone at hand to help with all your little requirements — holding the glass for you to have a drink, helping you to get comfortable in the bed, lifting the baby out of her crib at feeding time and so on — without needing to feel that you are endlessly asking the nurses for assistance. It will mean a great deal to both of you, too, to have the opportunity to share these first moments of being a family.

FOR YOUR BABY

Providing your baby is well, she will be tucked up in a crib next to your bed so that she is close to you. The first few hours, when you may be feeling tired and groggy, are an ideal time for the father to spend time with his baby, cuddling her and getting to know her while you sleep.

Initially the baby is cared for by the nursing staff, who will wash and dress her, change her nappy and generally keep an eye on her. As soon as you and the baby feel like feeding, ask the midwife to help you get the baby into a comfortable position. If you are breastfeeding for the first time, you will probably need help getting the baby latched on to the breast properly too. Don't be afraid to call on the midwife's expertise for this, as correct positioning of the baby at the breast is the key to successful pain-free breastfeeding (see Chapter 7). Likewise if you have chosen to bottle-feed, the midwife will advise you on the best way to go about this.

You will notice that the baby has a plastic clip at her naval and a short stump of umbilical cord. This will gradually dry out and fall off over the next few days, but it is important that the site is kept immaculately clean and dry to avoid any risk of infection. The midwife will show you how to do this.

Many babies are content to do little more than sleep or lie in their cribs, alert but happy, in this early time. Their entrance into the world is as exhausting for them, it appears, as it is for you, so they too like to rest and recover. Take advantage of this while it lasts — the peace is sure to be shattered before long. Don't be afraid to cuddle the baby, though, whenever you feel like it. Ask your partner or one of the nurses to lift the baby out of the crib and hand her to you when you want to feed her or just hold her close for a while.

Babies Who Need Special Care

If your baby is born prematurely or is small at birth or
there is some other complication, she may need to go into
the special care baby unit (SCBU) for observation or
possibly treatment. Babies born early often have difficulty
maintaining their body temperature and so have to lie
under special heaters to keep them at the right
temperature. They may also need help with feeding if they
are too small and weak to suck, and if they are very tiny or
unwell they may need help with their breathing.

It is quite possible after an emergency caesarean
section, especially if it has been performed because of fetal
distress during labour, for the baby to need to go to a
special care unit. Often this is purely so a careful watch
can be made on the baby's progress until the doctors are
confident that all is well, and it might only be for an hour
or so. In other instances, the baby may need more help for
a longer period and have to stay in the unit for days or
even, on rare occasions, weeks.

Some babies born by caesarean section experience
temporary breathing problems caused by inhaling some of
the amniotic fluid (the liquid surrounding the baby in the
uterus). This does not usually occur with a baby born by
vaginal delivery because the baby's chest is squeezed as it
passes through the birth canal. Fortunately most babies
who suffer this problem are perfectly all right after a
while.

If your baby has a low birth weight but is otherwise well,
she may be able to stay with you on the postnatal ward
and receive the specialist care needed there by your side.
For instance, if she is having a problem keeping warm, she
can be put in an incubator by your bed, so the two of you
do not have to be separated.

On the other hand, if the baby is very poorly at birth,
she may need to go to a unit offering intensive care. An
intensive care unit is similar to a special care unit but has
more sophisticated technology available to assist in
complicated or very specialised treatment. Not all
maternity hospitals have these facilities on the premises,

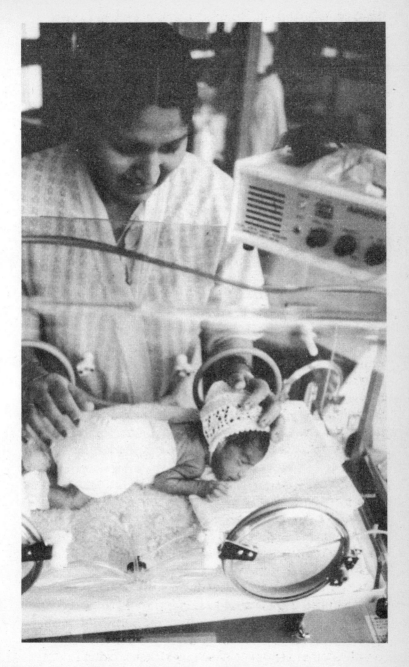

Baby in Special Care Baby Unit (SCBU)

in which case the baby would have to be taken to another hospital.

Having a baby that needs special care can leave you feeling shocked and overwhelmed with anxiety, especially if you are separated from your infant for any length of time. Some hospitals are sufficiently thoughtful to give a mother whose baby has to go to SCBU a polaroid snapshot of the baby to keep by her bedside, and this can do much to lessen the anguish of separation. If a photograph is not offered, ask the doctor if one could possibly be arranged for you. Equally important are explanations as to what is wrong and what treatment is required. Again ask the doctor to tell you exactly what the problem is, how severe it is and what the prognosis (likely outcome) is. There is nothing more anxiety-provoking than not knowing what is happening.

As soon as you are over the first after-effects of the operation, ask to be taken to the special care unit so you can see your baby, in a wheelchair if the unit is any distance away. The first sight of your baby may be both marvellous and shocking, particularly if she is hardly visible amongst all the equipment. The staff in these units are only too well aware of how desperately stressful a time this is for you and will do their best to be supportive. Ask them to explain the function of the pieces of machinery — don't be daunted by it. If you understand what the treatment is for and what exactly is being done you will find it easier to come to terms with it.

Even a baby in an incubator can be stroked and caressed through the portholes in the side and the contact will help both of you. More often than not you will be given every encouragement to breastfeed your baby if she can suck, and if she can't you can express your breastmilk, which can then be fed to her through her feeding tube. Most of all, try and spend as much time with her as you can, talking to her, stroking and touching her, simply getting to know her.

WHEN A BABY DIES

Despite modern technology and all the efforts of the medical staff, sadly some babies do still die. Such a loss is shattering and the parents will need to grieve for a long time before getting over it. Any parents facing a bereavement of this nature need special help and understanding to come to terms with what has happened. Often at such times the mind fills up with questions. Why did it happen? Couldn't anything have been done to save the baby? Could it happen again with another baby? A post-mortem examination may provide some of the answers to these questions. Talk the results through with your doctor until you feel satisfied with the explanations. Talk, also, to the doctors and nurses who looked after you and the baby, and don't be frightened to voice all the questions and concerns that crowd into your mind.

Nobody can take the pain of such a loss away, but the anguish may be eased by talking to other parents who themselves have suffered the death of a baby around the time of birth. Such help and support is offered by the Stillbirth and Neonatal Death Society (see useful addresses on pp. 173–5).

6
EARLY DAYS

FOR YOU

Regardless of what type of birth they had, most mothers
agree that the week after the birth of a baby, especially if
it is your first, is a time of extremes. As one mother
expressed it, 'It was rather like being an involuntary
passenger on an emotional and physical rollercoaster.' At
breakfast time you may be feeling on top of the world, only
to have plummetted to the depths by lunch; one moment
you feel supremely confident about handling your baby,
the next second you are in a blind panic about some minor
problem; one moment your excitement infuses you with
energy and you feel ready for anything, the next moment
you feel so weary you want to sleep for a week. The sheer
unpredictability of your emotions and sense of physical
well-being can leave you feeling panicky.

Fortunately it is also a time when you have plenty of
back-up support. Hopefully your partner will have time
now to devote to you and the baby, although it is
important not to forget that he too may be struggling with
the weight of responsibility imposed by his role as a father.
In the ward you are freed from mundane concerns such as
where the next meal is coming from and keeping the place
tidy. You also have the reassurance of expert advice and
guidance on hand as to the best way to care for your baby,
and immediate help available in coping with any problems
that might arise.

One tip mentioned by many of the women for coping at
this time is quite simple. Be kind to yourself. Accept that
the events of the last couple of days constitute a major life
experience for you — and your partner — and that it will
take time to adjust and settle down to your new life.
Remember too that, unlike most of the other mothers in

the ward who have given birth vaginally, you are not only adapting to a new role and trying to learn new skills, but you are also recovering from major surgery. Don't expect to do too much too early, but try at the same time to keep a positive attitude, doing a little more for yourself and your baby day by day. Let your own instincts guide you, both about what you feel up to tackling and on how you want to care for your baby.

Your physical state will be checked regularly by the nursing staff, twice a day in the initial period and then once a day later on. Your temperature and pulse rate will be recorded as usual, and a midwife will feel your abdomen to check that the uterus is contracting as it should. She will also keep a watchful eye on the wound to ensure that it is clean and dry and is not showing any signs of infection. If you have a drain in the wound this will be taken out on day two.

The nurse will also check your lochia (vaginal discharge) to see that it is normal. For the first few days the lochia will be quite profuse and bright red in colour, but gradually it will diminish in quantity and turn to a reddy-brown colour. You might notice that the loss increases and gets much brighter in colour after breastfeeding or any exercise. This is quite normal. However it is not normal for the lochia to start smelling unpleasant or for the flow to increase significantly for any length of time. If this happens you should alert the nursing staff, as it might indicate the presence of an infection. Don't be tempted to use tampons rather than sanitary towels as this will greatly increase the risk of infection.

A watch will also be kept on the condition of your breasts. These will become very large about three or four days after the birth, and may feel tender and hot as the milk comes in.

I woke up one morning and thought my neck was broken. No matter how high I tried to lift my head I could not see my feet because of these two huge solid mounds on my chest. *Kay*

Any discomfort should ease once the baby has started to feed regularly from the breast (see Chapter 7 for detailed discussion of breastfeeding techniques) and a good-fitting supportive bra will also help you feel more comfortable.

Each day that passes in this first week should mark a noticeable step forward in your physical recovery from the operation, until by the middle of the week you may well be on a par with some of the other mothers in the ward who had vaginal deliveries.

I used to sit cross-legged on the bed to breastfeed because it was the most comfortable way with my scar. I had just been thinking how lucky the woman opposite me was because, whereas I could hardly stand up, she could walk around the ward carrying the baby, when she came over and said how much she envied me being able to sit down. Her episiotomy stitches felt so uncomfortable that she even had to stand up to read the paper!

Caroline

Even so the caesarean mother does have extra physical handicaps to overcome, not the least being getting out of bed for the first time.

Getting on the Move

No sooner will you have surfaced from the initial after-effects of the operation than the nursing staff will be coaxing you into moving around as much as you can. Initially it is a good idea to do some deep breathing and to concentrate on exercising your legs and feet while you are still lying down as these will help your system get going again (see pp. 140–1).

Within 24 hours of the operation you will be encouraged to get out of bed. At a time when any movement, even laughing, causes you pain, the notion of standing upright might be too appalling to consider and you wouldn't be the first post-caesarean section mother to jump to the conclusion that all the nurses must be sadists for suggesting such an exercise. However, don't blame them. There are, in fact, pressing medical reasons for you to get mobile again as quickly as possible after the operation. First your circulation will have become sluggish as a result both of the anaesthetic and of lying still for so long, and this creates the risk of a number of complications, including the very serious one of thrombosis.

Second, becoming mobile again stimulates all the essential body functions back into full action, including breathing, digestion and bowels. This will speed up your general recovery and promote the healing process, and, although it might not feel like it immediately, this also means that you start to feel much better faster. A complete day-by-day programme of exercises specially designed for getting you back on the move is outlined in Chapter 9. You can also ask the hospital physiotherapist who visits you to advise on postnatal exercises, though be sure to remind her you have had a caesarean section, as not all exercises will be suitable for you.

One small word of warning. Don't try and get out of bed for the first time without assistance, or you might find yourself flat on the floor. Ask a nurse or your partner if he is available to help you. A stool by the bed will make it much easier. Take as much time as you want and move slowly, avoiding any twisting movements that might pull the wound. Also make sure your sanitary towel is in place as your vaginal discharge is quite likely to come in a rush as you stand up.

Set yourself a modest goal to start with, such as reaching the chair by the bedside, where you can sit while the nurses make your bed. You may be horrified by just how shaky you feel, not to mention how hot and sweaty you'll get from this minor exertion, but don't get despondent — it *will* get easier day by day. This is another reason for accepting the assistance of painkilling drugs in the first few days, so that the pain from the wound doesn't inhibit your movement any more than necessary.

When you have mastered getting out of bed and

standing upright, you can think about a gentle stroll to the lavatories. In case you feel dizzy from the effort it is advisable not to launch off down the middle of the ward where there is nothing to hang on to for support. Initially just aim to move from bed-end to bed-end. This is the time that every post-caesarean section mother can recall, when it feels as though you will never walk tall again.

I will never forget trying to walk to the toilets the first time. I felt dreadful. I didn't dare stand up straight because it seemed as though my stomach was going to split open, so I hobbled along like a little old woman, clutching my front. I had only shuffled about two yards when I felt so hot and dizzy that I had to stop and lean against the wall. 'I'm never going to be able to walk, again' I thought and burst into tears! Fortunately another woman in the ward walked over and gave me a hand. I told her I thought I'd never walk again. 'Yes, you will,' she said. 'I had a caesarean section five days ago and look at me!'

Dee

Although slouching over seems to be the instinctive response to the wound, it is in fact the worst thing you can do, because it pushes the weight of your internal organs against the scar, pulling it even more. Rest assured, the wound will not break open. Each layer has been stitched back together and there is absolutely no danger of tearing the stitches, so try to keep your posture as upright as possible.

Diet
For the first 12–24 hours your nutritional needs will be met by the drip in your arm which will supply you with water, sugar and minerals. Gradually you will start drinking, first water and then fruit juices and once you are taking in adequate quantities of liquid by yourself the drip will be removed. It is wise to avoid carbonated drinks as these will

only exacerbate any wind problems you might experience (see opposite page).

On day two you will be offered a light meal, usually consisting of soup and ice cream. Your initial intake must be fairly bland so that your digestive system is stimulated back into action gently. Once you have shown your system can tolerate a bland diet, and some rumblings and gurglings in the intestines testify that there is movement in that area, a more varied diet can be introduced, although the amounts of food should still be quite small.

As soon as your appetite indicates your digestive system is functioning properly again, try eating healthy foods — fresh fruit, vegetables, raw if possible, salads, wholemeal bread and so on. This will help ensure you don't fall prey to a common post-operative complaint — constipation. It is no fun straining with an abdominal wound! Unfortunately hospital food is not always the most inspiring, or, ironically, the most health giving, and many mothers confessed that they had encouraged their visitors to bring in picnics of more enjoyable foods.

Going to the Lavatory

Your bowel movements, or lack of them, will take on an alarming significance from about the third day after the operation. The nursing staff will question you closely and frequently about whether or not you have had one and, if the answer is negative, will threaten suppositories or an enema.

Often this concern with bowel movements is premature. Your system may well have been completely emptied prior to the operation and you will have consumed very little solid food in the first few days after it, so you simply will not need to empty your bowels for several days. It is, of course, important that your bowels get back into working order as you return to normal eating, but by following the tips given below this can usually be achieved without the trauma of intervention.

• Drink plenty of fluids (avoiding carbonated drinks).

- Move around as much as possible and keep up with your exercise programme.
- Ask your visitors to bring in fresh fruit, fingers of raw vegetables, nuts and perhaps even some prunes for you to eat.
- Eat muesli or a high-fibre cereal such as All-Bran for breakfast. If these are not offered on the hospital menu, ask your partner if he would bring supplies in for you.
- Add a couple of tablespoons of bran to your breakfast cereal or nibble bran biscuits.
- Avoid too many refined carbohydrate foods, such as chocolates, sweets and cakes.
- Use a high-fibre medicament (such as Fybogel) to add bulk to the stools, making them softer and easier to pass. Most hospitals have supplies of this type of medicament, or it can be bought in chemist shops.

If all this fails and you are getting uncomfortable, ask the nursing staff for a mild laxative. (You don't want to take anything too strong or it might pass to the baby through the breastmilk with catastrophic consequences!) And if that fails, ask for help!

The first bowel movement after a caesarean section can be extremely uncomfortable, as bearing down with your stomach muscles after abdominal surgery is bound to put a strain on the wound. The advice is to try and be relaxed and just let go. Concentrating on breathing exercises will help to keep your muscles relaxed and it can help to lean forward as you sit and hold your hands firmly over the wound. You could also try putting your feet on a low stool if there is one available so you are as close to a squatting position as you can manage; some women reported this position made it much easier for them the first few times.

Discomfort From Wind
Another potential hazard awaiting the post-operative caesarean mother is wind. Many women report some problems with wind, to a greater or lesser degree, about

the third day after the operation. Wind is the butt of many a music-hall joke but it can be very unpleasant and certainly no laughing matter for the sufferer. Some women even felt that the pain from wind was worse than the pain from the wound. Most hospitals have their own special cocktails, usually based on a mixture of ingredients including peppermint, hot water and a painkiller, for alleviating the discomfort of wind, so do tell the nurses of your distress. Alternatively ask your partner to bring in some anti-wind medicament, such as arrowroot, fennel tea or charcoal biscuits.

Getting on the move is undoubtedly the best way to combat wind pain, so try and walk around as much as you can. Following the exercise programme will stimulate the intestines into action and this will also help to alleviate the problem. Exercises which are particularly helpful are the deep breathing exercise (p. 141), the pelvic rocking exercise (p. 142) and exercise 10 (p. 147). Once your bowels are functioning normally the problem will disappear.

After-pains
In the first few days after the birth many women experience painful sensations rather similar to period cramps as the uterus starts to contract and return to its non-pregnant size (a process which takes about six weeks to complete). These after-pains may be particularly bothersome when you are breastfeeding, as the action of the baby feeding at the breast stimulates the release of a hormone called oxytocin which causes the uterus to contract. If you are finding it a problem, try taking a paracetamol 30 minutes before you start breastfeeding.

Feeling Low
It is the third day after the birth and you are beginning to feel better physically and to move around with much more ease. Your beautiful baby is asleep in her cot by your bed and all the visitors have cooed over her, much to your delight. Everything is roses— or is it? Why the tears that

well up at the most trivial hitch, the feelings of sadness and despair?

No one really knows why the so-called 'baby blues' set in, regardless of what type of birth experience you have had. More often than not they are explained away by reference to the rapid change in hormonal levels that occurs immediately after childbirth. What is known is that it is a very common emotional stage after birth — about 50 per cent of new mothers experience this low — and the staff of postnatal wards are perfectly used to seeing women weeping for no obvious reason about this time. Just because it is a common occurrence, however, in no way undermines the fact that it is very real and traumatic for the woman concerned, and she needs to be treated with special sympathy and understanding at this time.

Simply resting as much as possible can ease the intensity of the feelings. It may be worth seeing if your baby could be looked after in the nursery for a night, or even two, so you can get an uninterrupted stretch of sleep. Fatigue certainly exaggerates any problem and it is important not to expect too much of yourself too quickly. This is particularly true for you as a caesarean mother who has all the unpleasant after-effects of a major operation to cope with as well as getting to grips with the demands of your new baby.

> I thought I was never going to be able to cope. It hurt my wound even to hold the baby and I felt so tired all the time. Then I kept finding myself in tears; they would just gush out and even I didn't know what the matter was. I felt such a fool, but I couldn't help it. It all seemed too much.
>
> *Fran*

It may be taking a while, too, to reconcile yourself to the fact that your baby had to be born by caesarean section. Perhaps you feel cheated and angry about what happened and unable to accept that your expectations of the birth turned out to be so far from the reality. You may be particularly resentful if you had planned a completely natural birth. Or you may be blaming yourself, feeling you 'could have tried harder' in some way, or feeling you have 'failed' as a mother. You would not be alone with such feelings. Nearly all mothers whose babies have been born by caeserean section fall prey to such thoughts during this first week, as the realisation of what has happened sinks in.

If these feelings of bitterness and anger aren't to fester and manifest themselves later as depression, it is crucial you discuss with your doctor exactly why the operation was performed and whether or not any future baby would have to be delivered this way too. Understanding why the operation was considered necessary is one step towards accepting it, and once you have done that you may be free to stop looking back and start looking forward to life with your new baby. One important fact to grasp is that the type of birth you experience in no way dictates the quality of your mothering. Your relationship with your child begins at birth, but then unfolds slowly over time as you get to know each other. After all, a relationship that has to endure for years can hardly rest on the experiences of a few hours.

Talking about your feelings is an essential part of the healing process. Talk to the staff who are experienced, to other mothers who may be feeling the same or who at least know what you mean, to the doctor if you are worried about what has happened and want to know more, and, of course, to your partner so he can offer comfort and support. He, too, may be feeling shocked by what happened and would welcome the chance to talk it through so he can sort it out in his own mind.

Fortunately for the majority of women the baby blues pass off fairly quickly, in a day or so. If the feelings persist for much longer than that or grow in intensity, the problem may be more serious and you should seek specialised help (see pp. 130–34). Given the huge physical and emotional upheaval of childbirth itself and the awesome responsibility which rests on the shoulders of a new mother, the baby blues could be seen as a perfectly natural response to an extremely stressful situation. Perhaps the question should not be why do some women react in this way, but why doesn't every women feel like it?

Feeling Better

There are a number of practical ways you can make yourself feel better in these early days. Simply having a shower and washing your hair can give you a great boost. Some hospitals allow you to have showers from about the third day on and supply a little polythene apron for you to wear to protect the dressing. Other hospitals only allow washing at the basin or kneeling in a bath until after the stitches or clips have been removed. Once the stitches or clips have been taken out you can relax in a long hot bath. Don't forget to add plenty of salt to the water — this will help keep the wound clean and promote healing.

Making sure you are dressed as comfortably as possible can help to make you feel better too, or at least diminish some of the discomfort caused by huge tender breasts and a sore wound across your middle. Loose cotton nighties are recommended with large cotton, waist-high knickers underneath. Use stick-on sanitary pads so you don't have to wear a belt that will rub on the wound, and be sure to have nursing bras that fit well and offer good support. Rubber-soled slip-on slippers are a good idea so you don't have to bend down to put them on and there is no risk of slipping over on polished floors.

The removal of the stitches or clips can be a welcome landmark on the road to recovery. Many women are apprehensive about the procedure, but it should not be painful and the wound will feel much easier once the stitches or clips are out.

The nurses suddenly appeared in the ward pushing a trolley and a buzz went round — 'They're coming to take stitches out.' There were about five of us who had all had our operations on the same day so were due to have our stitches out at the same time. I had to be first, of course, much to my horror, but it really didn't hurt at all. The worst bit was getting the plaster off, but after that it just felt a bit ticklish. All that horrid tight feeling had gone too, so I felt much better afterwards.

Sue

When the stitches are removed depends on what the surgeon used to sew you up — clips are usually removed about day five, while stitches are usually left until about day seven. The scar will probably still look red and angry, but you can encourage healing by gently rubbing in wheatgerm oil or cocoa butter cream.

Take some time for yourself in these early days while you have the chance. At least in the ward you have the nurses who can watch over the baby, so you can take a stroll or read a book quietly or chat to the other mothers. Inevitably much of the talk in a maternity ward is about childbirth as everyone relates their individual experiences, but this can help you get your own experience into perspective.

Postnatal wards, unlike other wards in a hospital, are not peopled by the sick, so the atmosphere there is usually fairly jolly and relaxed — if rather noisy. Although the nursing staff give demonstrations on the various aspects of babycare, the opportunity to watch other mothers handle their babies can be very useful, too, if only to reassure you that all first-time mothers find it just as nerve-racking as you do.

There was an Indian lady in our ward who had had her first baby. Every day she was visited by her mother who, she told us, had brought up 14 children in all. If any of us had got a problem or were worried about our baby for some reason, we would creep over during visiting hours to consult her. There was something very reassuring about listening to someone who had looked after so many babies — and survived it.

Francis

The stream of visitors that appears at the news of a birth can be a source of great pleasure and entertainment. Your morale can get a dramatic boost from hearing everyone praising your baby — and you — to the skies. Sit back and enjoy it all — life will return to normal soon enough. Be careful not to let it get too much, though. You may be taken aback by just how tiring visitors can be, so try to keep it to one or two people at a time.

Most of all be sure there is plenty of time for you to be together as a family. If this is your first baby, adjusting to life as a family can take time — and practice. Not only do you both have to get to know someone who is a complete stranger, but you also have to adjust to seeing each other in your new roles as parents. The more time and effort you invest in this now, the stronger will be the foundations on which the family rests. The sheer joy at just being together as a threesome is often reward enough for all the hard work and pain.

If you already have children, their excitement at the arrival of a little sister or brother can be very infectious. Try to ensure that they have every opportunity to come to the ward and share in the welcome party.

FOR YOUR BABY

A careful watch will be kept on your baby by the nursing staff in this first week of life. The site of the umbilical cord is cleaned and checked daily to see that it is healing properly and that there is no sign of infection. Her nappies are scrutinised to ensure that her bowel movements are normal. For the first two or three days she will pass a greenish-black, rather sticky substance called meconium which accumulated in her stomach while she was in the uterus. Then, as feeding becomes established, this is replaced by stools that are much looser and bright yellow in colour, with a fairly strong smell if she is breastfed and firmer and a slightly darker yellow if she is bottle-fed. In the first few weeks the stools are passed frequently.

Her weight is also checked daily. Don't be alarmed that her weight drops initially. This is perfectly normal and is a consequence of the meconium being cleared from her system. After about a week her weight should start to pick up again and increase steadily from then on.

Many newborn babies spend much of the time in this first week asleep. When awake and not feeding they are often content to lie in their cots or in their mothers' arms, just looking around. Despite appearances to the contrary, a newborn baby's senses are highly developed even at this stage. Their sense of smell, hearing and vision are already at work exploring the immediate environment. Your baby will be particularly drawn to the human face and by holding her up close to your face she will soon learn to recognise you. She will also learn your special smell — researchers believe it is the odour of the individual breastmilk the baby picks up on especially. She will also be tuning in to all the noises around her, particularly the sound of your voice and the father's, so talk to her whenever you are holding her.

Babies are born equipped with a number of reflexes, one of the most important being the rooting and sucking reflexes. If you brush a finger against your baby's cheek, she will instantly turn her head towards the finger and open her mouth. This is the reflex you use to attach the baby to the breast if you are breastfeeding. (Full details of breastfeeding are given on pp. 110–19.) She will also automatically start sucking once she has latched on to the breast. Other reflexes are lost after the first weeks, such as the grasp reflex — a baby can grip tightly not only with her hands but also with her feet — and the stepping reflex — if a newborn is held in an upright position, she will make stepping movements with her legs. Sometime in the first few days a paediatrician will check that your baby shows all these reflex responses.

Jaundice

This is a very common complaint among newborn babies, especially if they were born pre-term. It usually appears about the third or fourth day after the birth and manifests itself as a yellowing of the skin and the whites of the eyes. Generally it is very mild and disappears without treatment in a week or so.

If the condition is more severe the doctor may treat it with phototherapy, which speeds up the breakdown of the yellow pigment. The baby is put naked into a special cot with bright violet lights overhead and a soft mask is placed over her eyes to protect them. In some hospitals the phototherapy unit can be placed next to your bed, but more often than not it is in a special care unit. Treatment in this way can last several days but you will be able to continue breastfeeding as normal during breaks in the treatment. If this fails to clear up the jaundice an exchange blood transfusion may be required. This is where some of the baby's blood is drawn off and replaced by fresh blood so that the pigment is removed from the bloodstream.

With most cases of jaundice the only drawback is that the baby may be more lethargic than usual and this can mean that there are difficulties in getting breastfeeding established. However as the baby's condition improves, so her desire to feed will increase and the problem should rectify itself.

GETTING READY TO GO HOME

Both you and the baby will be given a thorough medical examination before leaving the hospital to go home. The baby will be examined by the paediatrician, who will listen to her heart and check all her reflexes. He or she will also check her limbs and her genitals and test for any sign of dislocation of the hips. This last test involves moving the baby's hip joints quite forcibly in a circular motion, and every baby protests at such treatment. However it is an important test because any dislocation can be treated relatively easily and with minimum distress to the baby, providing it is diagnosed early on.

A blood sample will also be taken to test for a rare biochemical condition called phenylketonuria. The test is called a Guthrie test and involves taking samples of blood from the baby's heel. Again, although briefly distressing for the baby, it is crucial that the test is done because if the condition is left untreated it could lead to brain damage.

An appointment will be made for you to have a postnatal check at the hospital in six weeks time and you will be told about the medical back-up from the community midwife and then the health visitor that you can expect when you get home. The nursing staff will also give you details about how to register the birth, which must be done before the baby is six weeks old.

Sometimes before you leave the ward either the doctor or one of the nurses will advise you about contraceptive methods. If you are like most mothers at this time, sex will be the last thing on your mind! However, the important point to absorb is that you can get pregnant again before you have your first period after the birth, even if you are breastfeeding. So when you and your partner do feel that way inclined you will need to take precautions.

With your head buzzing from all this advice you are now ready to set off back into the big wide world, a little sore but accompanied by the most precious of bundles.

7
FEEDING YOUR BABY

One of the questions you are asked on your first visit to the antenatal clinic is whether you have thought about how you want to feed your baby, by the breast or by the bottle. Feeding is a surprisingly emotive topic and often people feel very strongly about it. Some mothers insist that the only way to feed a baby is by the breast and anything else would mean depriving a baby of the best start to life. Others claim that the whole idea of breastfeeding appalled them and their babies thrived perfectly happily on formula milk taken from a bottle.

Forty years ago there was almost no question about how a mother fed her newborn; every mother breastfed unless there was a medical reason that prevented her from doing so. In the late 1950s there was a dramatic swing away from breastfeeding to bottle-feeding and, despite the recent publicity in favour of breastfeeding, this swing has by no means been reversed.

The most important point is that the decision how to feed your baby is yours — you should decide what you think would be the best for the two of you. However it is a choice that should be based on knowledge and not just on hearsay.

Whichever way you choose to feed your baby, feeding should be a time of closeness for the two of you — a time for emotional as well as physical nourishment, when you can enjoy simply being together.

BREASTFEEDING

The first point to make clear is that just because you have to have your delivery by caesarean section does not mean that you cannot breastfeed your baby. Even if you have felt too unwell for the first day or so after the operation to want to feed, breastfeeding can still be successfully established, with a little guidance, encouragement and — very important — patience.

Many of the mothers who had their babies by caesarean section spoke highly of the emotional, as well as physical, benefits of breastfeeding. They claimed that for them breastfeeding their babies helped erase some of the deep disappointment felt when the birth had not gone as they had planned. They also felt it enabled them to regain a sense of harmony with their babies after the trauma of the delivery, and restored their confidence in their own ability to mother — something that in many instances had been seriously undermined by the need for a medical delivery.

But there are other equally persausive reasons for trying to breastfeed your baby.

- Breastmilk contains exactly the right nutritional balance to ensure a newborn baby grows healthy and strong.
- The colostrum — the liquid that flows in the first few days before the milk comes in — lines the baby's gut and helps protect her from infections such as gastroenteritis.
- There is evidence to suggest that breastmilk also offers protection against such allergic diseases as eczema and asthma, as well as providing resistance to many childhood illnesses like ear infections, coughs and colds.
- Breastmilk is easily digested and breastfed babies rarely suffer from constipation because the stools are much softer and therefore easier to pass.
- Once breastfeeding is established it is very easy in practical terms — no messing about with sterilisers or

worrying about being caught away from home without a bottle.

- From the mother's point of view, breastfeeding helps her body to get back to normal more quickly. It encourages the uterus to return to its pre-pregnancy size and uses up any excess fat she may have put on during the pregnancy.
- If your baby was born before full term there is an extra reason why breastmilk is best. Research has shown that the mother of a pre-term baby produces milk which is much higher in ingredients vital to the development of the smaller baby.

Breastfeeding is a completely natural simple action. However it is crucial to bear in mind that, in contrast to the baby, who is born with the instinct for feeding from the breast, for the mother breastfeeding is a learnt skill. She has to acquire the ability by being shown how to do it and then experimenting until it works.

It is interesting to note that chimpanzees who are born in captivity do not know how to breastfeed and have to be shown how to suckle their babies. In the wild they would have learnt this behaviour by observing other female chimpanzees nursing their young. Similarly many women these days have not handled a baby or watched another woman breastfeed until their own infants are thrust into their arms. Consequently they have simply no experience of the mechanics of breastfeeding.

I had this dreamy picture in my mind while I was pregnant, of my baby sucking contentedly at my breast. I just assumed women were born knowing how to breastfeed and thought it would be like falling off a log. How wrong can you be! For a start he wasn't interested and then when he finally was hungry I got such sore nipples I could hardly stand it. Fortunately the midwife in the hospital showed me what I was doing wrong and I was able to position him better so it didn't hurt. He seemed happier too and from then on it was a great joy for both of us.

Judith

So don't be surprised or disheartened if, in the beginning, it takes a little time for you to learn the knack of breastfeeding and for the two of you to work out a successful feeding routine together. Offer your baby the breast as soon as you feel like it after the operation. Initially she might not be interested in feeding but might just nuzzle the breast and then be happy to be held close. Gradually her appetite will increase, but the first few attempts can be viewed as practice sessions, for you to discover a comfortable way to feed and to ensure the baby takes the right part of the breast into her mouth, and for the baby to learn that sucking at the breast means she will get milk so she is eager to feed.

Normally the milk comes in on the third or fourth day after the birth — up until then the breasts produce colostrum, a creamy-looking liquid which is rich in protein and antibodies (protection against infections) and therefore of great benefit to the baby. Occasionally women who have had a caesarean section find that their milk is a little slower coming in, say on the fourth or fifth day, especially if they have been unwell after the operation and therefore not able to get up and move about, or there was a delay in putting the baby to the breast in the beginning.

As the milk comes in your breasts may become large and heavy, and possibly feel extremely uncomfortable. Much of this discomfort can be eased by breastfeeding and wearing a comfortable supportive cotton nursing bra. If your baby is in a special care baby unit, express milk with a breast pump until the baby can feed from you. Sometimes the breasts become quite huge, and this has the effect of flattening the nipple. If this happens, it may be necessary to express some milk before trying to get the baby to latch on. You might also find that you are leaking milk everywhere and need to change breast pads frequently to keep yourself clean and dry.

Unfortunately this rather difficult and uncomfortable time often coincides with the period known as the baby blues (see pp. 100–103). It is now that the support of your partner and the help of the midwifery staff can be invaluable. Try and bear in mind, too, that this messy awkward phase will pass in a day or two as the rhythm of the baby's demands and your supply settles down.

The Importance of Position

The position for breastfeeding is important in two respects: first, it is crucial you are comfortable while you are feeding for the let-down reflex to work (the reflex by which the milk comes down from the breast to the nipple); and, second, the baby must be correctly fixed on the breast for her to feed successfully.

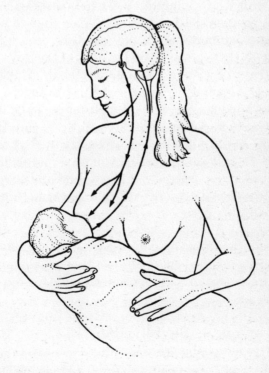

The let-down reflex

There are a number of ways you can position yourself and the baby to avoid any painful pressure on your wound, and it is a matter of experimenting to see which one is the easiest and most comfortable for you. Here are two that many mothers have found useful.

- **Position 1**. Lie on your side with pillows up against your back for support. Lay your baby on a pillow, with her feet pointing up towards the top of the bed and her mouth by your nipple. If the nipple touches the side of the baby's cheek she will open her mouth, turn towards the breast and latch on. When the baby has finished on that breast and has let go of the nipple spontaneously, you can ease her, on her pillow, a little way across your chest, so enabling her to latch on to the other breast.
- **Position 2**. If you prefer, you can breastfeed in a sitting position. Sitting cross-legged on the bed with pillows to support your back is one way, or alternatively you can sit on the edge of the bed with your feet on a stool, or in an upright chair. Make sure you aren't leaning backwards as this will flatten your breasts and make it more difficult for the baby to latch on. Equally important, check you are not slouching forward or you will end up with backache. Lay the baby on a pillow (or pillows if you need more) on your lap to avoid any pressure on the wound and support her across her shoulders with your forearm, being sure not to flex her neck.

If you find it painful to hold her on your lap, try lying her on a pillow by your side with her feet tucked under your arm. With the same arm support her shoulders and head so she can reach the breast.

The Technique — Step-by-Step
Once you and the baby are in a comfortable position, the next crucial stage is to ensure that the baby is latched on to the breast correctly. This simple manoeuvre is the key

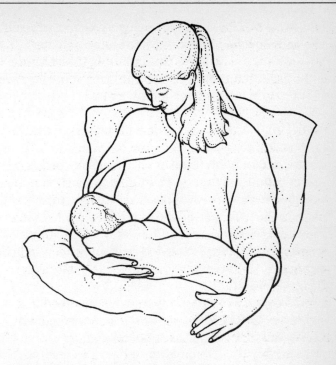

Breastfeeding in a sitting position

to trouble-free breastfeeding, but it is also one where the
standard advice given is often confusing.

The first step is to stimulate the baby's natural reflexes
for feeding. These are her rooting reflex, as it is called, and
her sucking reflex. By gently touching the baby's cheek
with the nipple the baby will be stimulated to turn her
head towards the breast and to open her mouth in
preparation to grasping the breast — this is the rooting
reflex in action. Once the baby has taken part of the breast
into her mouth, the touch of the nipple on the **roof** of her
mouth stimulates the sucking reflex and she will start to
feed.

The advice given to breastfeeding mothers on attaching
the baby to the breast is often phrased as 'the baby should
take as much of the areola (the brown area around the
nipple) into her mouth as possible'. This is, however,
slightly misleading, because as you look down at your baby

on your breast, the part of the areola visible to you is the area on the top of the nipple, whereas in fact the area that is critical for correct fixing is the area **below** the nipple and the surrounding breast tissue. So the correct position best achieved by feel rather than by sight. Dr Woolridge of Bristol University, who has been studying the anatomy of infant sucking with Chloe Fisher, a midwife of some 30 years' experience, describes the process like this: 'the mother must first "plant" the lower rim of the baby's mouth well *below* the nipple, and them almost "fold" the breast into the baby's gaping mouth'. This way the baby takes in what Chloe Fisher calls a 'hunk' of breast with her lower jaw and tongue.

A common misconception is that the nipple is synonymous with the teat on a bottle. This leads many mothers to believe that a baby should take just the nipple into her mouth, in the same way as a bottle-fed baby takes the teat on the bottle. This is a completely false notion. Unlike the teat of a bottle, the nipple does not contain any milk; it is merely the channel through which the milk is drawn from the breast. The 'teat' that is created by the baby sucking at the breast is, in fact, made up of the nipple *and* some of the surrounding breast tissue. Consequently, as Dr Woolridge points out, 'The "teat" is about three times as long as the nipple at rest.'

When your baby is fixed correctly on the breast, you will find that even vigorous sucking doesn't cause you any pain, or make the nipples sore. Your baby will feed calmly, following the familiar pattern of phases of sucking actively interspersed with pauses. She will let go of the breast spontaneously when she has finished and you can then offer her the other breast. Do not worry if she doesn't want to feed any more this time; just offer her this breast first at the next feed. Your milk supply adapts to the baby's demands after about 24 hours, so any discomfort caused by her not feeding from both breasts is short-lived.

Feed as often as the baby shows a desire to do so, and allow her to stay on a breast until she breaks off herself. The old-fashioned advice of timing feeds from each breast

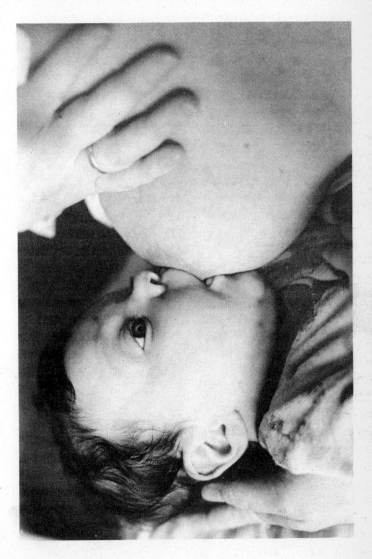

Baby incorrectly latched on for breastfeeding

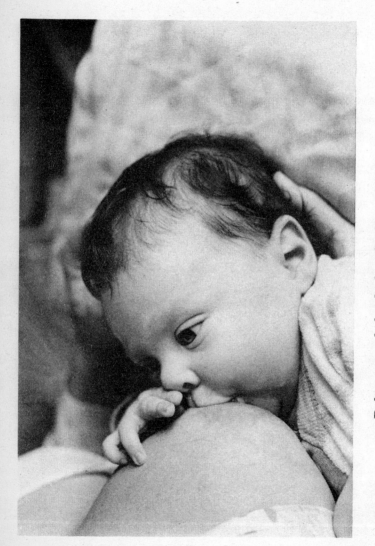

Baby correctly latched on for breastfeeding

has now been shown to be incorrect. The foremilk that comes when the baby starts feeding is more dilute than the more nutritious, thicker hindmilk. By switching the baby from breast to breast after a certain amount of time rather than by her own indication that she has finished means not only that she doesn't get enough of the hindmilk, which she needs for her growth, but that she is also getting an excess of lactose, the natural sugar found in breastmilk, which can lead to problems with wind and diarrhoea. Result — an unhappy baby, and an unhappy mum. Leaving the baby to come off the breast herself when she is satisfied overcomes this problem.

Further Tips

Your diet is important while you are breastfeeding. Eat small, frequent meals to keep up your energy levels and drink plenty of fluids. Many mothers sang the praises of drinking Guinness while breastfeeding, not least for its effect of keeping them relaxed so the let-down reflex worked! (Interestingly some recent research has shown that it is not the alcohol that has the beneficial effect here, but the beer itself.)

Getting sufficient rest is another key factor in successful breastfeeding, so make sure you take every opportunity to put your feet up.

Advice on breastfeeding can be obtained from organisations such as the National Childbirth Trust and the La Leche League — see Useful Addresses on pp. 173–5.

BOTTLE-FEEDING

Most authorities are agreed that breastmilk is the healthiest food for a newborn baby. However if you decide to bottle-feed for medical reasons or just from personal choice, you can rest assured that modern formula milk offers a good alternative to the real thing and there are a great many babies that have thrived on this style of feeding.

The non-medical reasons why women choose to bottle-feed are numerous. Some simply find the idea of breastfeeding offputting; others attempt to breastfeed but run into problems and decide that they just can't cope and so switch to bottle-feeding.

One of the advantages of bottle-feeding is that someone other than the mother can feed the baby occasionally, giving her the opportunity to rest and recuperate. This is where many fathers come into their own.

Fiona was very low after the operation and it was decided that the baby should be bottle-fed. At first I was as upset as Fiona about this, but I soon began to enjoy feeding times because I could feed our baby. It was wonderful to hold her in my arms and see her contentment as she drank from the bottle. Then I'd wind her over my shoulder and as often as not she would fall asleep in my arms. It gave me enormous pleasure — I know how women feel now — and also a sense of being a real parent, because I could satisfy her needs all by myself. Fiona soon reconciled herself to it when she saw how eager the baby was for the bottle and how much I enjoyed it too.

Michael

Formula milk is cow's milk that has been modified so that a baby can digest it happily. There are numerous brands on the market and it is best to ask your doctor or midwife to recommend one. It is important to follow exactly the instructions on how to make up a feed, and again this is something you will be shown by the midwives in the postnatal ward.

Scrupulous attention to cleanliness is vital because the bottle-fed baby is more at risk of infection. Breastfed babies receive antibodies in their mother's milk which help guard against infection, but as yet nobody has found a way of putting such protection into formula milk. This means that all the bottles and teats must be thoroughly washed and sterilised after use. Milk residues are especially receptive to bacteria which would make the baby ill if they weren't killed off by sterilising.

Finding a comfortable position for feeding is just as important with bottle-feeding as for breastfeeding. Sitting on the bed or in a chair and laying the baby on pillows on your lap, so the pressure is taken off your wound, is perhaps the most comfortable position.

Don't rush the feed, but cherish the relaxed time together. It is equally possible to feel close and warm while bottle-feeding as with breastfeeding.

8
HOME AT LAST

If this is your first baby, the real time of adjustment comes when you go home and life returns to its more familiar setting. The first realisation is that your whole world is different now, and no matter how prepared you thought you were for this change, the reality of it can hit you like a bombshell. You are not only you now, you are also a mother. Your partner is not only your friend and lover, but also a father. There aren't just two of you to care for, there are now three — and one of those is astonishingly demanding. Some new mothers adjust quickly and relatively easily to their new roles; others take longer and find it decidedly traumatic.

> After about the fourth day in the hospital, when I had begun to feel more mobile and the wound was easier, I longed to go home. I thought it would be wonderful to be in my own home with my baby and I kept on nagging the doctor to let me go. He was reluctant at first, saying it was better to stay in and rest for a while longer, but I had become obsessed with going home. Finally he discharged me on the sixth day and my husband came to collect the two of us to take us home. I was so excited. But by the time we drew up outside the house the baby was crying and I was crying because the movement of the car hurt my wound. I walked in the front door and was hit by this huge wave of panic. I suddenly realised that it was all down to me now, no nurses to ask for advice, no other mums to chat with, just me. I have never felt so small, so alone and so unable to cope before. I nearly ran back to the car and asked my husband to take me back to the hospital.

Fran

If this is not your first baby, you have the advantage of having worked through this period of shock before, of knowing the ropes. Even so, this time you have a new dimension to cope with — being physically debilitated after the operation. You may be surprised to find that the usual demands of your family can seem just too much in the first few weeks, until you start feeling physically stronger and your energy returns.

For the next few weeks, it is important that you — and those around you — respect the fact that you have had major surgery, not just given birth which is exhausting enough, and that your body has to have the chance to heal. You may well find that you get tired quickly and this can be very demoralising at a time when you feel under pressure to do so much. The simple answer is don't try to do more than you can. Conserve your energies for your baby and for recuperating. Let household chores drop to the bottom of the list of priorities, and if possible delegate them to other willing hands for now. If your partner, friends or relatives are happy to wait on you, enjoy it. The time will be shortlived and the usual daily routines will start soon enough, so there is no need to feel guilty about making the most of it now. If you don't have anyone around who can help you, ask the midwife or your health visitor how you can go about getting a home help supplied by social services (see p. 50).

Your physical recovery is crucial to your general sense of well-being, so it is worth paying some attention to looking after yourself as well as your baby. Any negative feelings will become exaggerated if you let yourself get rundown. Getting over the physical impact of pregnancy and birth is hard work for any mother, but it is an even harder uphill struggle for a caesarean mother. Your wound will be sore and will limit what you are able to do comfortably for quite a while. However, be patient — every day will bring a noticeable improvement as the wound gradually heals, your strength returns and you all settle down to life as a family.

Eating well is one important way of getting your body's

strength up and this is particularly important if you are breastfeeding. Make sure your diet contains plenty of fresh fruit and vegetables, wholemeal bread and grains, and protein. If there isn't anyone to help prepare food for you and you want a quick snack, try an easy pick-me-up drink. Put a glass of milk, a banana, one egg, two teaspoonsful of honey and a sprinkling of brewer's yeast in a liquidiser and blend for a few seconds. It's fast but nutritious and will help to keep you going.

Keep up your exercise programme too (see Chapter 9). This is the time when it is only too easy to let your exercise routine flag, and yet it is also the time when you can make the most progress. Your wound will be easier now and allow you much greater freedom of movement to tone up your muscles again. It might be easier if you set a certain time aside each day for doing your exercises, say during the baby's first sleep in the morning. It might seem like a chore to start with but you will probably be pleasantly surprised to find that exercising leaves you feeling *more* energetic and alert.

Be very careful, however, not to put too much strain on your wound in these first few weeks. In particular avoid lifting anything heavy, whether it be a basket of washing or your toddler. Also most doctors recommend that you don't drive for at least three weeks after the delivery as this will also pull your abdominal muscles.

Equally important as exercise is rest. The advice 'get as much rest as you can' may ring a little hollow at a time when you are lucky to get more than four hours' sleep at a stretch. If you have other young children as well, it is essential to have help for the first couple of weeks or fatigue will overwhelm you and hinder your physical recovery. Grab any and every opportunity for a nap or just to sit for a moment with your feet up. Don't think, 'I'll just clean the kitchen . . . put the washing on . . . tidy up', or whatever, when the baby drops off to sleep. Go straight to bed and do the same. Perhaps your partner could take on one of the night feeds occasionally, so you can get a restorative stretch of uninterrupted sleep. You can express milk for a relief bottle and keep it in the fridge if you are breastfeeding.

BECOMING A PARENT

Almost all new mothers experience a range of emotions, ranging from exhilaration to panic, utter contentment to despair, for the first couple of months. About the only variation on this theme is the intensity with which you feel them. One thing that can influence these feelings is knowing and accepting that you have to *learn* how to be a good mother. You are not innately endowed with the knowledge simply by virtue of being a female member of the species. All learnt skills take time and practice to acquire, so don't expect too much of yourself, too quickly.

Faced with the full responsibility of looking after Clare I suddenly realised I didn't know a thing. I had had very little contact with babies until we had our own and I simply didn't know what to do half the time. Jeremy had to bath her for the first four weeks because I was panic-stricken that I would drop her in the bath. I used to feel myself go tense at the first sound of her cry, too. On top of that, I felt much more tired than I expected to and my scar really ached by the end of the afternoon. The first month was hell in a way, but things are improving now. I feel more confident about looking after Clare and seem to understand better what she needs. I feel stronger too and walk around for longer before I notice the scar hurting. I just never imagined it would take so long for everything to fall into place and felt very inadequate and disappointed in myself in the beginning.

Jane

This learning process is just the same for the father — he too has to acquire the skills attributed to a good parent. There is perhaps not so much pressure put on him while he is learning his new role — he is not expected to achieve so much so fast, while the woman is expected to take full responsibility for the care of her baby from the first moment — but it can still be a difficult, if exciting, time of adjustment for a man too.

An essential part of learning to be a mother is realising that, despite it being your most demanding and rewarding role, it is only one element of your character. You are still a person in your own right who deserves time to and for yourself. Resentment can build up surprisingly quickly if you allow yourself to be completely taken over by your baby, so do try to find moments for yourself — take a long, relaxing bath, sit with your feet up and read a book, do something that is just for you.

As well as enjoying each other as a family, be sure to make time for just you and your partner now and then too. Ask a trusted friend to babysit and go out for a meal, see a film, do whatever you enjoyed doing together before your baby was born. Keeping in touch with the bits of you that were there before you became parents is vital, or you might find they are in danger of being completely swamped.

Re-establishing your sexual relationship is important here. Initially this may not involve sexual intercourse, although physically you can make love as soon as you feel you want to after the birth, once your vaginal discharge or lochia has dried up. But don't worry if you do not feel like sex for the first couple of months — or even more — after the arrival of the baby. Many women — and men — find they are just too exhausted and tense to be very interested in much sexual activity until life has settled down a little. Also the soreness of your wound can put you off love-making until the scar is well-healed. However this does not mean you cannot be warm and gentle towards each other and take pleasure from other forms of close physical contact.

On Your Own
The first day your partner goes off to work and you are left alone in the house for a whole day of being a mother on

your own can be an alarming time. It is important to keep up your contacts — or establish new ones — outside the house. If you allow yourself to become socially isolated, any problem is at risk of getting out of proportion. Talking to other mothers, whether they are just learning like yourself or experienced at the task, can help keep worries and concerns in perspective.

Often women who have worked before having their babies simply don't know any other mothers locally. If you are in this position, ask your health visitor if she knows of any groups you could join. Alternatively organisations such as the National Childbirth Trust or the Meet-a-Mum Association may be able to put you in contact with other mothers in similar situations. If you particularly want the opportunity to talk about your caesarean section and to hear how other mothers coped with this type of delivery, you could see if there is a caesarean support group in your area (see useful addresses on pp. 173–5).

MEDICAL BACK-UP

For the first few days after leaving the hospital you should be visited on a daily basis by a community midwife. She will check that your wound is continuing to heal and that your body generally is returning to normal. The soreness and redness of the wound will gradually diminish, and as it heals it may well become rather itchy. The midwife should be able to recommend creams or a powder to help calm the itchiness if you find it a problem.

The midwife will also examine your baby, including measuring her weight, to ensure she is developing satisfactorily. If you have any worries or queries about the baby's progress or your own health, she should be able to advise you. Your GP may also visit you to check on your and the baby's progress.

When your baby is about 10 days old, the midwife will hand over your care to the health visitor (although in some areas the midwife will continue to visit for a longer period). A health visitor is a fully qualified nurse who has received

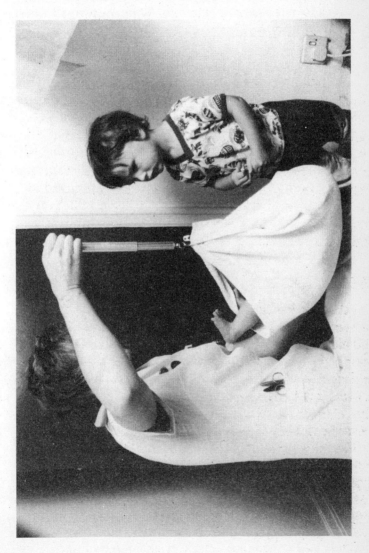

Midwife weighing a baby at home

extra training so she can advise on family health. She will visit you at home until you are up to getting yourself and your baby to the local baby clinic. Again, should you have any worries or problems, do talk to your health visitor as she is trained to be able to help you. Your contact with the health visitor will continue, in fact, right up until your child goes to school.

Six weeks after the delivery you will have an appointment at the hospital for a postnatal check-up. This should be a fairly thorough physical examination to ensure that you are recovering fully from the birth. You will be weighed, your blood pressure will be measured and a sample of your urine will be analysed. The doctor will check that your wound is healing properly and feel your abdomen to see that the uterus is back to its non-pregnant size. He or she will also carry out an internal examination and probably do a cervical smear test at the same time.

This is also your chance to voice any concerns or queries you may have, either about your recovery or about the operation itself. If you feel that you were never given a satisfactory explanation as to why the operation was performed, now is the time to ask. It is important you clarify the reasons for your caesarean section in case it is a problem that could recur and mean you would have a caesarean section delivery next time too (see Chapter 10).

FEELING DEPRESSED

The vast majority of mothers have moments in these first few months when they feel down and unable to cope. Such times can be seen as inevitable and natural when all the changes that follow childbirth are taken into account. At a physical level a woman's body undergoes rapid and extensive changes following birth; while at a social level she has to learn to handle effectively a whole new set of demands and play a previously unrehearsed role as a mother. Perhaps even the much-publicised role of modern woman as 'superwoman' has a part to play. So much is expected of women these days, not least by women themselves, and trying to fulfil unreasonable expectations can take a heavy toll.

Negative moods that appear and then disappear fairly quickly can be seen therefore as par for the course, but feelings of lethargy, despair, panic or anger that persist for any length of time are not. If this is how you are feeling, ask someone for help. Don't try to struggle on, hiding the tears and the fears, but talk to your partner, your health visitor, your GP. The important point is that help is available if you ask for it. Just talking to someone sympathetic can bring enormous relief.

It has become apparent over the last few years that far more women than was ever previously suspected fall prey to postnatal depression. Postnatal depression should not be confused with the baby blues which affect many women shortly after the birth of a baby and disappear after a couple of days or so (see pp. 100–103). Unlike the baby blues, postnatal depression might not surface for weeks, even months, after the birth. Typical symptoms are tearfulness, feelings of inadequacy and being unable to cope with the baby, overwhelming fatigue and lethargy, poor appetite and difficulty sleeping. These feelings can continue for a considerable time if the woman is not given support and help. Fortunately the old attitudes of 'she ought to pull her socks up' and 'she's got a lovely baby, so what's the matter with her' are no longer so common, and a woman who is suffering in this way can usually expect to be treated with sympathy and understanding by the medical profession.

As far as medical research has been able to discover, a woman who has had a caesarean section is no more likely to suffer from postnatal depression than a woman who has had a vaginal delivery. It is common, however, for women who have had caesarean sections, elective or emergency, to take time to reconcile themselves to the nature of their deliveries. And certainly if any of the negative feelings that surface are not examined and dealt with effectively, there is the risk they might fester and result in serious depression.

Any woman who has invested a great deal of time and effort in planning and preparing for a natural birth, only to have her expectations dashed by requiring a caesarean section at the last moment, is undoubtedly going to feel disappointed and upset. Disappointment is one of the reactions most frequently mentioned by caesarean mothers — disappointment in the birth, in themselves, and sometimes even in their babies. The latter response is by no means unique to caesarean mothers, though. A great many mothers feel disappointment and detachment in relation to their babies, and are horrified to find they can harbour such emotions. Yet it is in many ways a natural reaction. It is inevitable that over the long weeks of the pregnancy a woman will build up in her mind's eye an idealised picture of this new life growing inside her. After the birth, disillusionment can set in if the real baby bears little resemblance to the imagined one and the woman finds herself confronted by a complete stranger that she has to get to know and learn to love.

In the late 1970s great emphasis was placed on the notion of bonding, a concept which seemed to suggest that something akin to emotional cement was produced in the first few hours after the birth, binding the mother to her child for all time. The implication from this was that those mothers who were unable to be with their babies in those first crucial moments, perhaps because they were recovering from an anaesthetic after a caesarean section or because the baby needed special care, were inevitably inhibited in their ability to love and cherish their babies. This idea caused caesarean mothers in particular considerable anxiety.

Fortunately the theory has fallen into disfavour recently as experience and medical research have exposed the flaws in it. The relationship between a mother — and a father for that matter — and a child begins after birth, but it continues for years to come. During that time it grows and develops, and is moulded by the many events and interactions within that family. Common sense alone would indicate that such a relationship could not be a static affair, determined solely by the contact — or lack of it — of the first few hours of a child's life.

Anxieties and negative emotions such as these affect many women after a caesarean section, so, first, rest assured you are not the only one who has ever felt this way. Second, bear in mind that many mothers feel like this in the first few months of new motherhood, even if they had a 'normal' vaginal delivery. Third, if you talk to someone and share your feelings, it helps to get them into perspective and any problems can appear more manageable. Finding out if there is a caesarean support group in your locality would be a good start, so you can share your worries with other mothers who will know exactly what you are talking about.

I was all right on the outside, smiling face and the doting mother, but inside I felt such despair. I couldn't escape from the feeling that I had failed because I had to have a caesarean section. It made me feel as though I wasn't a proper mother or something, because I hadn't been able to give birth normally. Fortunately a friend of mine introduced me to another woman in our town who had had a caesarean section a few months earlier. She had felt so strongly about it that she had set up a support group for caesarean mums in our area and I was able to go along there. We all found it a great help, being able to meet regularly in each others' houses and chat about our babies and how we were feeling. It certainly gave me a lot of confidence and I came to realise my baby's birth had been more of a triumph than a failure!

Sarah

A common misconception held by people who have not experienced caesarean birth first hand is the idea that it is an easy option compared with labour and vaginal delivery. Such thoughtless and ignorant comments have caused many a caesarean mother considerable distress and can exacerbate any feelings of failure that they may have been harbouring. If someone says this to you, you should remind yourself exactly what you have been through: you have had to undergo major surgery, endure post-operative pain which can be as intense as that experienced during vaginal delivery and cope with the physical stresses of post-operative recovery which are generally much more demanding than those experienced by mothers after a normal birth, while looking after your baby as well as any other mother. Decide for yourself if all that can be described as the easy option and then you should be feeling rightly proud of your achievement!

If talking to a sympathetic person doesn't alleviate the feelings of depression, it is crucial to seek specialist advice. Do tell your health visitor or your GP about your problem — they will be able to offer you help. Organisations which also might be able to advise you are the Association for Post-natal Illness and the National Childbirth Trust (see useful addresses on pp. 173–5).

YOUR BABY

Coming home is a time of adjustment for your baby as well as for yourself. She has to get to know a whole new world, with a new range of noises, smells and sights, even get used to a new cot, so it may take a few days for her to settle down too.

Simply spending time together and getting to know each other should be your main aim in the first few weeks. If you try and organise the practical details into easy routines that minimise effort, you will be free to enjoy your baby. For instance, ensure that you have all you need for nappy changing downstairs as well as in the baby's bedroom so you don't have to wear yourself out traipsing up and down stairs every half hour.

Over the next few weeks you and your baby will adjust to each other and life together will develop a more relaxed pattern as a consequence. Your confidence as a mother will grow as you find that you understand what your baby's needs are and get know how to satisfy them. Your baby will also come to recognise you as the most important person in her life and respond accordingly, making you feel much more rewarded for all your efforts. Around five weeks of age she will give you her very first smile — a timely reminder of why you wanted a baby so much.

9
EXERCISING FOR RECOVERY

Establishing a routine of planned exercise and relaxation after the birth of a baby is important for all mothers, but for you as a caesarean mother it is the key to a speedy and successful recovery. If you can regain your sense of physical well-being as quickly as possible you will be much better equipped to meet the demands of your new role and so be a relaxed, confident and fulfilled mother.

If this is your first baby you may be surprised and bewildered by the body you now have. No one expects to return miraculously to their pre-pregnancy figure the minute the baby is born, but the sight of the flabby bulge where you hoped there would be flat tummy muscles can be rather a shock.

Why doesn't anyone ever tell you how horrible and fat you are even after the birth. I couldn't believe it. I felt like I had lost an enormous amount of weight but when I stood up for the first time and looked down I saw this great lump — I still looked six months pregnant! It was a terrible shock.

Jennifer

The muscles of the abdomen will have stretched considerably to accommodate your growing baby during the preceding nine months and will now be weak and slack. These muscles will regain some tone naturally, but they will also need help from gentle exercising to return to their former strength. As a caesarean mother you will also have all the problems of your scar to contend with. In the early days just getting out of bed may seem such an effort that the idea of exercising fills you with horror.

Don't despair. You will gradually be able to move around with more and more ease. After the first few days you will find it easier to stand up straight while walking, and slowly the tummy bulge will diminish as the uterus contracts, although it does take about six weeks for the uterus to return to its normal size. What you have to realise now is that not only do you have to meet all the demands of your new baby — and as you have probably already discovered, no one can truly forewarn a new mother about just how demanding this little bundle can be — but also that you have got to put some hard work and effort into yourself if you are going to get back to your old self.

Every woman recovers from the trauma of birth at her own pace, so do the exercises when and as often as you feel able to, and do not judge your progress by comparison with other mothers. If you were fit before the birth you will be able to move on to the more strenuous exercises quite quickly. If you had a difficult pregnancy that meant you had to rest much of the time, or had a long labour before the caesarean was performed, it will obviously take longer for you to feel up to doing very much exercising.

It is best to do a few exercises often rather than having one concentrated burst that might lead to strained muscles. As you do more exercises, you might notice an increase in your vaginal discharge, but this should not mean there is a problem. (However if you notice clots in the discharge, you should inform a nurse.)

The time bands given for the exercises in the following pages are meant as rough guidelines only. Work through them at a rate that suits you, and if an exercise hurts, don't do it. Stay with the less rigorous exercises until your muscles tell you they can cope. It is well worth trying to retone your muscles as quickly as possible so you are in peak physical condition to make the most of your new role, but it is equally important not to push yourself too hard or you will only strain the muscles and overtire yourself. If you are at all worried about how much exercise to do, talk to your doctor or the hospital physiotherapist about it.

If you have put off exercising because it all seemed too much in the early days, start today. It is never too late. And you will feel well rewarded for the effort when you notice how much fitter you are and how much more energy you have for looking after and enjoying your baby.

EXERCISES

Doing gentle movements from the day of the operation onwards will help your scar to heal, your muscle strength to return and the pain to go away. Be careful not to do too much too soon, but do try to set yourself little tasks or goals for each day. The first day after the operation just getting out of bed to a nearby chair, or going to the loo with the help of a nurse, seems enough. By the next day you should feel a little better, so try to persuade yourself to take short walks up and down the corridor every two or three hours, in addition to your trips to the lavatory. Then maybe on the third and fourth day you will be up to finding the odd job to do around the ward, such as filling the water jugs or refreshing everyone's flowers.

It might feel a dreadful uphill struggle to move around in the first few days, especially if you had a general anaesthetic, but the sooner you can make yourself get on the move, the quicker you will heal and the better you will feel.

I would recommend getting up as soon as possible after the caesarean to prevent stiffness and to accept the pain-relieving drugs on offer to enable you to move around more easily.

Angela

The exercises given below start on day one, taken as the day after the operation. If you have had an epidural anaesthetic you may feel up to doing some of the exercises a few hours after the operation, but most women find that the first 12 hours or so are spent in a state of euphoria over their new baby and post-operative shock. As soon as you feel able to, try doing the first exercises to help your system back into action. Build up gradually by increasing the number of times you repeat a particular exercise, and the number of exercises you do each day.

Note: after the birth of a baby you should never lie on your back with straight legs and try lifting both legs together nor should you attempt to do sit-ups with straight legs. Both these movements are too strenuous for this postnatal time and you could do yourself a serious injury if you attempted them.

DAY ONE

After a caesarean section your circulation becomes sluggish as a result of the anaesthetic and from lack of mobility, so the first goal is to improve the circulation to prevent complications such as thrombosis developing. Try and do the following exercises once an hour while you are restricted to bed. Once you are up and about they can be stopped.

Exercise 1 — Feet and Ankles
Lie flat on your back, with your legs stretched out straight. First bend your feet up towards you, then stretch them down towards the bed in a pumping action. Grip with your toes. Repeat this movement for about 30 seconds.

With your feet a little apart, circle each foot, first to the left ten times, then to the right ten times.

Exercise 2 — Legs
Sit up in bed, supported by your pillows, with your legs stretched out straight. With your toes pulled upwards, tense your thigh muscles and try to press the back of your knees against the bed. Hold while you count to five, then release the muscles.

Exercise 3 — Buttocks

Now do the same tensing and relaxing process using the
muscles of your buttocks.

Exercise 4 — Breathing and Coughing

If you have had a general anaesthetic you may find you
feel very chesty and want to cough because the lungs have
filled up with mucus, but coughing hurts your scar. One
way of minimising the pain is to sit up with your shoulders
crouched forward and your forearms cuddling your
tummy to support your scar — you can hold a pillow to
your tummy if this helps — then take three or four breaths
and 'huff' the air out of your lungs rather than trying a
normal cough.

Deep breathing exercises will also help to clear your
lungs. Lie on your back with your legs slightly bent and
the soles of your feet flat on the bed. Place the palms of
your hands on each side of your ribcage. Breathe in slowly
and deeply through your nose. You should feel your
ribcage expand beneath your hands as the lungs fill up
with air. Now relax and breathe out as much of the air as
possible through your mouth, tightening your abdominal
muscles at the same time by pulling them in towards your
back. Breathe in and out naturally, then repeat the deep
breathing. Practise this exercise several times a day.

DAY TWO

Keep up the exercises from day one and try the following.

Exercise 5 — Pelvic Floor

Even though you have not had a vaginal delivery, the
muscles of the pelvic floor will have become stretched
during pregnancy. If they are not strengthened again, it
can lead to a number of problems in the future including
exertion incontinence, vaginal slackness and even prolapse
of the uterus. This is why this is one of the most beneficial
exercises you can do at this time — and for ever more! Try
to do the exercise several times a day — while sitting

feeding the baby, resting on your bed or, when you get home, standing at the sink or talking on the telephone.

Tighten the muscles round your anus, vagina and urethra, hold for a count of three then relax. Repeat this exercise ten times.

When you are able to get yourself to the lavatory you can check how well this exercise is working. As you are urinating, tense your muscles in that area and stop the stream for a moment, then relax and continue. This action uses the same muscles and will give you some idea of how weak or strong they are now.

DAY THREE

Repeat exercise 5 and try the following.

Exercise 6 — Pelvic Rocking

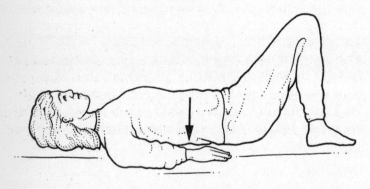

This exercise starts to strengthen your stomach muscles and also helps to ensure that the lower part of your back does not stiffen up.

Lie on your back with your knees bent and your feet flat on the bed. Squeeze your buttocks together, gently pull in your stomach muscles and press the small of your back against the bed. Hold for four seconds, then let go slowly and completely.

As you feel stronger you can increase the length of time you hold the position, up to ten seconds.

DAY FOUR

Repeat exercises 5 and 6, increasing the time spent on each one, and attempt the following.

Exercise 7 — Hip Hitching

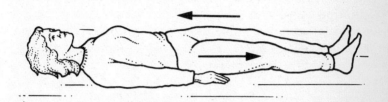

Lie on your back with your legs stretched straight and your arms by your sides. Pull up your left hip at the waist so that the left leg looks shorter than the right. Repeat with the right leg. Do this exercise five times for each leg.

Exercise 8

Lie on your back, with your knees bent and your feet flat on the bed. Your arms should be at your sides. Now press your elbows into the mattress for some leverage and lift your head to look at your knees. Relax for a moment, then repeat. Start by repeating five times, then build up to ten times.

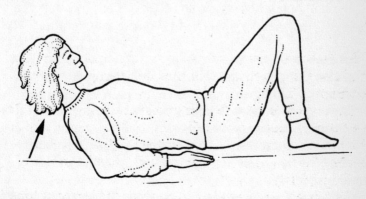

Exercise 8, part 1

143

(As you gradually regain your strength, stop using your arms to help you. Rest your hands on your thighs, tighten your tummy muscles and lift your head to look at your knees.)

Now in the same position, stretch your right hand down as far as you can towards your right heel, then stretch your left hand down towards your left heel. Repeat five times each side.

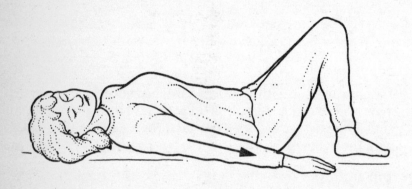

Exercise 8, part 2

DAY FIVE

Movement should be generally much easier now, so try to keep up exercises 5 to 8 and add the following routine.

Exercise 9

Sit up on the edge of your bed, checking that your back is straight. Put the fingertips of each hand on your shoulders and circle your elbows forwards five times, then backwards five times.

Keeping your hands on your shoulders, now try to twist your body first round to the left (only go as far as feels comfortable), then round to the right. Move your head so that you can watch your elbow as you turn, and take care to keep the movement as smooth as possible. Start by

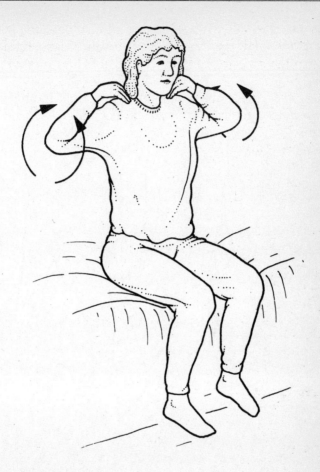

Exercise 9, part 1

doing the exercise five times in each direction and
gradually build up as the movement becomes easier.

DAY SIX UNTIL YOU GO HOME

The length of time you stay in hospital will depend on how
you and the baby are progressing and the policy of your
particular hospital. Most doctors recommend that you
stay in hospital for seven to ten days — you have, after all,
had major abdominal surgery as well as given birth.

145

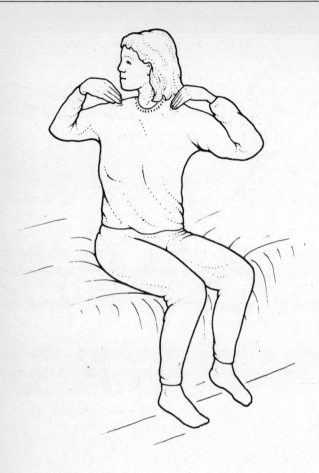

Exercise 9, part 2

Over the next few days continue with exercises 5 to 9 and, as you feel the strength returning to your muscles and the pain from the wound lessens, try some of the more adventurous routines given below. As always, do not push yourself too hard and if you feel any twinges of pain, stop and concentrate on the gentler movements for a little longer.

Exercise 10

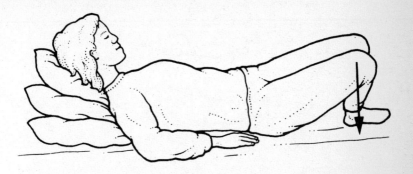

Lie on your back with knees bent, legs together. Avoiding any jerking movement, let the weight of your knees take your legs over to the right. Lift them back to their original position, then let them drop over to the left. Repeat ten times to each side.

Still lying flat with your knees bent, lift your head and shoulders off the pillow and try to touch your knees with your head. Hold for the count of four, then slowly lower your head and relax. Repeat five times to start with, building up to ten times as the abdominal muscles strength.

Exercise 11

Either on your bed or on the floor, get on all fours and 'wag your tail' — twist your hips to the right and move your head and shoulders towards them, then do the same to the left. Repeat ten times.

Staying on all fours, pull in your tummy muscles as tight as you can so that your back arches. Hold the position for a count of five, then release the muscles and lower your back to the horizontal. Repeat ten times.

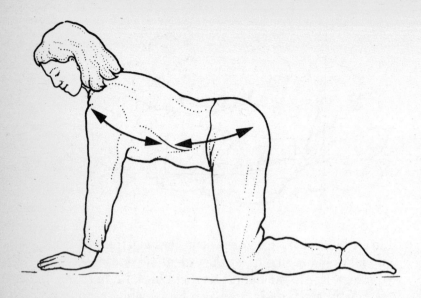

Exercise 11

Exercise 12
You might find that it is possible to lie on your front again now (for the first time in quite a few months!). For the most comfortable position, place one pillow under your tummy and one under your head and shoulders. Lying on your front is supposed to help your uterus return to its normal size. While in this position, try to tone up your bottom area by repeatedly squeezing and releasing your buttock muscles.

Exercise 13
Stand at arm's length from a wall, feet together, hands flat on the wall level with your shoulders. Keeping your back straight let yourself fall forwards as you bend your arms, then push yourself back up straight again. Repeat ten times in the first instance, working up to twenty.

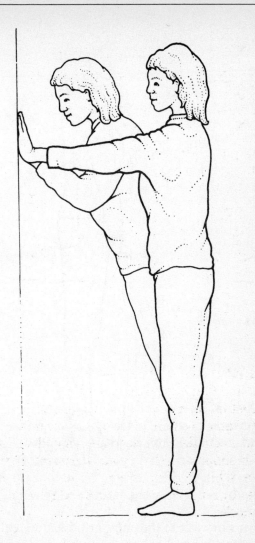

Exercise 13

Exercise 14
Holding on to the back of a sturdy chair or table, rise up on to tiptoes, lower slowly back on to the flat of your feet, then roll back on to your heels and lift your toes off the floor. Relax and repeat ten times.

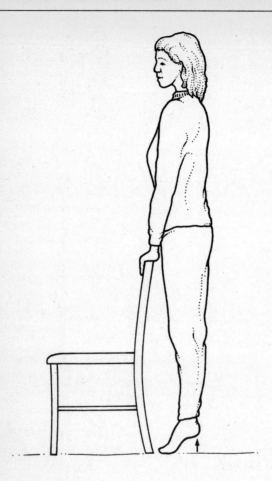

Exercise 14, part 1

Now turn sideways to the chair or table and, balancing yourself with your hand on the chair, swing your inside leg backwards and forwards, gradually swinging it higher and higher. Make sure you keep your back straight. Turn round to face the other way and repeat the movement using the other leg.

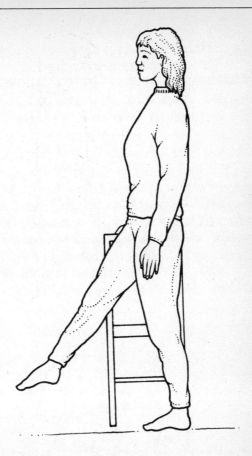

Exercise 14, part 2

AT HOME

This is the danger time for letting your exercise routines slip. You would not be the first mother who in the excitement of being at home again, plus the effort of establishing new routines for the household around the demands of its latest addition, found that exercising slipped to the bottom of the priority list. Yet it is in these early weeks that you will notice the greatest drain on your energy levels and when exercise and planned relaxation are most beneficial in continuing your recovery to meet these new challenges.

Take all the help that is on offer at this time, whether from your partner, friends, relatives or home helps. This leaves time for you to concentrate your energies on the baby — and on yourself. Putting effort and time into exercising now means that you will be well on your way to being back to normal by your six-week check-up. It does not take very long — 10 to 15 minutes a day should be plenty. A good time for exercising is in the morning, perhaps while the baby is having his morning nap, because, believe it or not, you will probably feel more energetic after exercising than before!

Do not forget to continue with your pelvic floor exercise (exercise 5) as many times a day as you remember. Also repeat exercises 10 to 14 and progress to the following routines as you gain in strength and flexibility.

From week three onwards try the following:

Exercise 15

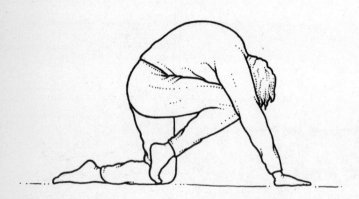

Exercise 15, part 1

Kneel on all fours. First bring your right leg forward and try and touch your forehead with your knee. Then stretch your leg out behind you and hold for a count of three. Return to the all-fours position and relax. Now do the same action with the left leg. Repeat five times with each leg.

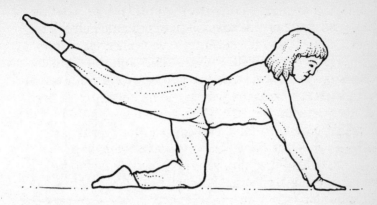

Exercise 15, part 2

Exercise 16

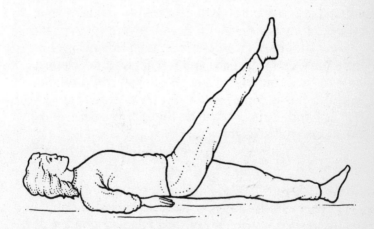

Lie on your back on the floor with your legs stretched out straight in front. First lift the right leg up as high as you can and then lower it slowly to rest on the floor. Repeat with the left leg, ten times in all. (*Don't* try to lift both legs together, as this will put too much strain on your abdominal muscles.)

Then from week four onwards you could try the next three exercises.

Exercise 17

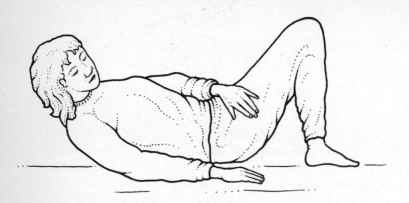

Lying on your back, with your knees bent, feet flat on the floor, tighten your abdominal muscles and stretch your right hand across your body to reach the outside of your left thigh, lifting your head up to watch your hand at the same time. Hold for a count of four, then slowly lower yourself back on to the floor and rest for a while. Repeat using your left hand to reach across to your right thigh.

Once this has become fairly easy, try to reach your knee with your hand. Finally try to do the exercise with your legs stretched out straight.

Exercise 18

Standing with your left side against a convenient wall, feet slightly apart, check that your back is straight, tummy in. Then lift your right arm up over head and stretch the fingers to touch the wall. At the same time, stretch your left arm down the side of your left leg. Make ten smooth rhythmical thrusts. Now turn around and, standing with your right side to the wall, repeat the exercise.

Gradually you should be able to reach the wall with ease. As this happens, stand further away from the wall, so that you have to stretch more.

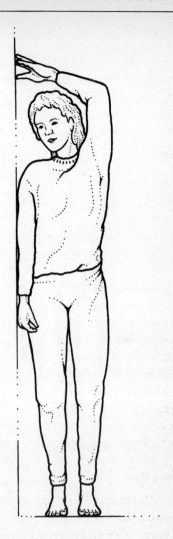

Exercise 18

Exercise 19

As well as concentrating on getting your abdominal muscles back into shape, it is worth spending time on toning up your pectoral muscles too.

Sit on a firm chair, back up straight, feet a little apart and firmly on the floor. Grasp your forearms with the opposite hands and lift your arms so that they are at chest

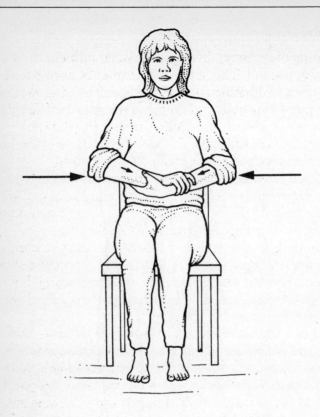

Exercise 19

level in front of you. Keeping your grasp firm, push your hands repeatedly up towards your elbows. You should feel your pectoral muscles contract and relax.

This exercise can be done as often as you can find a moment in your day to practise it.

As you gradually feel fitter and more energetic you might like to join a postnatal exercise class. The National Childbirth Trust run classes in some areas (check with your local branch) or your health clinic may organise classes. This way you have group support to help you through the exercises and the added bonus of a chance to chat to other mothers.

POSTURE

During pregnancy, there are two main influences on the way you stand. The first is the pregnancy hormones which produce a softening effect in the ligaments, the second is the increasing bulk and weight of the growing baby. Unless a woman takes care to watch her posture while she is pregnant, she will often find that by the time of the birth she has developed a very poor posture indeed.

Once you are up and about after your caesarean section, it is important to check your posture and correct it if necessary. At first, standing up will be very painful and you will be tempted to lean forward, clutching your tummy, as you shuffle along. In fact leaning forwards is the worst thing you can do as it throws the weight of your internal organs against the scar, thus increasing the pressure on it. It might feel as though the stitches are going to rip open, but, be assured, they won't.

When you get home from the hospital, check your posture in a full-length mirror. Stand sideways to the mirror and check the position of your shoulders, your tummy and your bottom. How do you look? Are you all slumped up, shoulders drooping, tummy sticking out, knees bent? Or do you sag forwards, tummy caving in?

Now imagine you are a puppet worked by strings. One of the strings is attached to the top of your head and someone is pulling it up. Feel your back straighten and lengthen. Let your shoulders relax downwards — often when people are concentrating on standing up tall, they pull their shoulders backwards in sergeant-major style. This is not correct. Just let your shoulders relax, with your arms hanging loosely by your side. Feel your neck lengthen. Now pull your tummy in and tuck your bottom in at the same time. Relax in the position. Take a deep breath and feel your chest expand outwards. Try and remember how it feels now, the sensation of standing tall effortlessly.

At regular intervals during the day check your posture — while you are out shopping, pushing the pram, nursing your baby, washing up at the sink, wherever and whenever

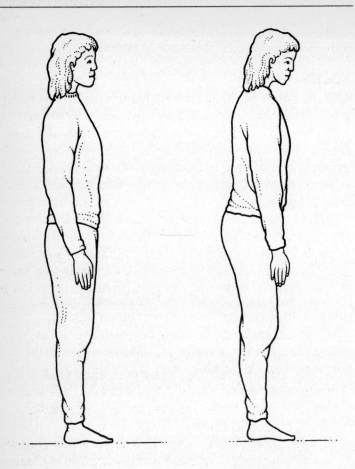

Good posture   **Bad posture**

something jogs your memory and reminds you about it. Imagine being a puppet again and recall the sensation of standing up straight. Correct your posture accordingly. You will find it becomes second nature quite quickly.

Correct posture is not only good for your body, reducing the risks of strain and injury, especially to the back, and generally helping to minimise the effects of tension; it is also good for your morale. Someone who stands well and easily has a natural air of confidence, which impresses itself on those around them, helping them to feel more relaxed. What is more, by adopting a confident posture you will help yourself feel more in control.

Backache

Unfortunately backache is very common after the birth of a baby — as indeed it is during pregnancy. There are many reasons for this, although faulty posture is one of the main culprits. By correcting your posture regularly and gradually improving your muscle tone by following the exercise routines, you will hopefully find that any back pain disappears.

Many of the movements that you will be called upon to do in a normal day can potentially strain your back if done incorrectly. Check that you are not making any of the common mistakes that can lead to back strain and injury.

- Are you sitting properly? The temptation is to slump in a soft armchair, but this can be very bad for your back. Opt for a chair which gives your back firm support and allows your feet to be flat on the floor and your knees bent at right angles.
- If you are breastfeeding, are you tending to sit crouched over your baby? Again this can put undue strain on your back. See the correct positions for feeding given in Chapter 7.
- Do you have to bend over when you are changing your baby's nappies? If you use a chest or table to change her nappies on, it should be at about waist height, allowing you to stand up straight. Or choose a lower surface so that you can kneel down to do the job. This applies equally to bathing and dressing the baby.
- Do you always remember to keep your back straight and bend at the knees when lifting a heavy object or your toddler, so that your legs rather than your back take the strain? If you do decide to carry shopping home, divide it into two carrier bags rather than one heavier one, so that you can balance the load.
- Do you find that you are having to stoop forwards when pushing the pram? Check that the handle is not too low for you.

- Do you get backache after carrying your baby in the
  sling? Perhaps she is simply too heavy for you to carry
  this way and you would be better off finding another
  means of transport.

I had always liked the idea of carrying my baby around
in a sling, close to me all of the time. One day I caught
my reflection in a shop window — tiny me (I'm only 5
feet 2 inches and weigh 7 stone) with this great bump on
the front. I could see how much I had to lean back to try
and compensate for Tom's weight on my front — it was
no wonder I had backache! The next day he was in his
pram. I missed having him close, but I didn't miss the
pain in my back going away.

Margaret

RELAXATION

It is not just exercise that is important in this postnatal
time. Plenty of rest and relaxation are also crucial to
recovery and should be incorporated into your daily
schedule. As every mother knows, this is easy advice to
give but it is often extremely difficult to put into practice.
Again, as with exercising, if you can find the time and the
energy to try to set up a relaxation routine, the benefits
will be immediate. It will help you become aware of areas
of your body where tension is causing stiffness and
possibly pain, so you can be on the watch for anything that
might exacerbate this strain and lead to injury. Most of
all, it will help you simply to feel much better. A few
moments of relaxation can loosen the muscles in your
neck, shoulders and face, leaving you feeling calm and
refreshed, and perhaps ward off the tension headache that
had been looming. A tension-free body is altogether better
able to withstand the effects of stress, so you not only feel
better in the short-term, but are also laying the
foundations for future health.

These first weeks at home with a new baby can be a

very tense time — lots of new skills to learn, new routines to be established, loss of sleep to be borne. Indeed, sleep will inevitably become a very precious commodity until the baby settles down to some sort of routine and a sense of day and night (this is usually after about the sixth week). Consequently it is worth trying to learn the art of napping to see you over this time and to ward off complete exhaustion. Try to nap whenever there are a few spare moments of peace, say for 15 minutes after each feed.

Although you might think that relaxation is something that happens naturally, given the right conditions, it does in fact have to worked at. If you watch a cat or dog move from tense alertness to complete relaxation in a couple of seconds, you can see that it is a natural, instinctive response for them. Unfortunately human beings seem to have all but lost this capacity for natural relaxation and instead have to learn techniques to help them gain a state of relaxation. Often men and women do not recognise just how tense they are becoming, until the aches and pains start or the outbursts of temper or despair appear. Learning ways of relaxing now can do much to counter the unavoidable frustrations and exhaustion of early parenthood.

Deep Relaxation

This form of relaxation is particularly valuable for banishing tension from your body and calming your mind. It is an excellent way to wake up (if this is a luxury you are allowed, as opposed to being dragged from your slumbers by the cries of your infant) and, more especially, an ideal way to ensure peaceful, refreshing sleep at night.

Lie flat on the floor or on your bed, legs out straight in front of you, a little apart, feet flopping outwards, arms by your sides with the palms up. Start by having a good long stretch, down to your toes and your fingertips. Then let your limbs feel loose, close your eyes and concentrate on your breathing. Breathe in (not too deeply) then let the breath out very slowly and, as you breathe out, let all the tensions in your body flow out with the air. Breathe like this five times, concentrating on letting the tension go with the out breath. Now breathe normally.

- Always start with the same muscles, say your toes and ankles. Think about relaxing them, let them feel loose and heavy (if they roll outwards that is a good sign that you are relaxing).
- Now focus on your leg muscles — think about relaxing them. (If you find this difficult because you do not know what it feels like for muscles to be relaxed, try tensing the muscles first, then letting them go.)
- Now move on to your tummy muscles. Feel your back sink into the floor or bed as you relax.
- Relax your shoulders, feel them drop downwards. Now your arms and hands; let the fingers feel floppy and curl slightly.
- Think about your neck and your head; let the muscles relax. Release the tension in your neck muscles and let your head feel heavy.
- Relax your face muscles. Smooth your forehead, let your jaws loosen and your lips relax.
- Breathe evenly and concentrate your mind on the feelings of warmth and heaviness in your limbs. Stay in this relaxed state for 10 minutes.

Initially you might find yourself getting fidgety after a few minutes. If this happens, don't struggle to maintain the position but stop the exercise and try again later. You will gradually be able to hold the relaxed state for longer periods.

When you stop, don't jump up immediately. Take it very gently. Breathe in deeply and stretch all your muscles, then sit up slowly.

Five-minute Relaxation
By adapting the technique for deep relaxation, you can do a five-minute routine at odd moments during the day — say mid-morning, in the afternoon and in the evening. It will help dispel fatigue and revive flagging spirits.

- Sit in a comfortable chair that supports your back well and allows your feet to rest flat on the floor. Allow your hands to rest easily in your lap.
- Close your eyes and concentrate on your breathing, taking a breath in and letting it go slowly. Feel all the tension in your body flow out too. Breath calmly in this way for a moment.
- Starting with your feet, consciously relax each part of your body in turn.
- Now try to empty your mind of all thought (concentrating on a sound way off in the distance sometimes helps with this).

Rest in this relaxed state for a couple of minutes, then open your eyes, take a few deep breaths and you will be ready to tackle anything.

Quick Relaxation

Use this technique if you feel yourself getting worked up or in a panic about something — perhaps the baby will not go to sleep and you are feeling close to the end of your tether. It might help reduce the build-up of tension and anxiety, and once you are relaxed your baby probably will be too.

- In your mind say to yourself firmly, 'Calm down now.'
- Breathe in, then release the breath very slowly. As you breathe out, consciously relax your shoulders and neck (the most common point in the body for tension to accumulate).
- On the next slow out-breath, relax your face — smooth away the frown, release your jaws (you will probably find you had been clenching your teeth without even noticing), relax your mouth.
- Breathe in, and as you breathe out say to yourself 'I am relaxed. I am calm.'

MASSAGE

Have you noticed how much you cuddle and stroke your baby? This touch is calming and reassuring to the infant, and it can be equally rewarding for you. Scientific studies have shown the many physical benefits of massage — how it reduces blood pressure, improves the circulation, lowers the pulse rate, relieves tired and aching muscles. But massage also has a psychological impact. It can soothe someone who is anxious and ease away the tension in their muscles, leaving them revived and refreshed.

It is also a way of conveying care and affection. And at a time when there seems little energy left over from the demands of the new baby, it can be a way of having loving but non-sexual physical contact between you and your partner.

Obviously you do not want anyone massaging your tummy when the scar is still painful, nor will it be comfortable enough to lie on your front for a full back massage for quite a while, but the most common tension spots that can benefit from massage are the shoulders and neck, the face and the hands. All these areas can be massaged by your partner with you sitting comfortably in a chair.

We used massage in the hospital to help me with feeding. I think that the nurses were a bit amazed if not rather shocked, until they saw how it worked. After about the third day after the caesarean operation I felt weepy and tense and was having real trouble feeding. Mike came in at visiting time and said, 'It's the let-down reflex, you know. You're too tense.' So he took up position behind me and started massaging my neck and shoulders. It felt wonderful. After a bit I put the baby to the breast while he kept massaging my shoulders. It worked a dream and the baby had her best feed since she was born. I can recommend it to anyone if they feel themselves getting worked up.

Juliette

HINTS AND TIPS

- Every time you stand up or are walking around, check your posture and correct it if necessary. Say to yourself 'Stand up tall.'
- Push yourself a little, but never too much.
- Do your pelvic floor exercises every day — for ever and ever.
- Make time every day for your relaxation routines.
- Take a brisk walk (or two) every day.
- Check that your pram handle is at the right height for you, that you are not having to bend over to it.
- Do not carry your baby in a front sling if he is too heavy for you.
- Don't carry heavy shopping. Do it piecemeal rather than all at once, unless you have someone who will carry it for you.
- Don't pack your supermarket shopping into a big box at the bottom of the trolley. You've got to lift it out.
- Smile. It helps you to relax your face and other people smile back, making you feel better!

10
THE FUTURE — ANOTHER CAESAREAN?

If, when you have had a caesarean section, the first question that springs to mind is 'Why?', the second question is nearly always, 'Will I have to have a caesarean section next time too?'

Fortunately the attitude of 'once a caesarean, always a caesarean' is not so common in medical circles as it once was. The phrase was originally coined at a time when surgical techniques were in their infancy and the risk of the scar rupturing during labour was very real. However, since the use of the lower segment incision of the uterus (see p. 75) became common practice in caesarean sections, the risks of rupture of the scar in a subsequent delivery have been considerably reduced. So the good news is that many more women can — and do — go on after a caesarean section to have their next baby successfully by vaginal delivery.

Some — although very few — obstetricians are even prepared to let a woman who has had a classical incision (a vertical incision in the upper segment of the uterus) have a 'trial of labour'. This change in attitude results from the fact that concerns over a spontaneous rupture of the classical scar are based on very old data, from a time when caesarean section was often accompanied by sepsis (infection) which further weakened the scar.

Remember, if you have had a caesarean section already and hope to try for a vaginal delivery next time, it is not the visible scar on the abdomen that affects the decision

167

but the scar inside on the uterus. These two incisions are not always done the same way. If you are unsure what sort of uterine incision you had (as opposed to the abdominal incision), ask for your medical records to be checked.

Although the danger of rupture of a previous uterine scar is now very low, the risk is still present. Consequently it is very unlikely that a woman who has had a caesarean section for a previous delivery will be allowed to have a home birth. In hospital, though, the woman's progress in labour will be closely monitored and if, in the rare event, a rupture does occur, then the signs and symptoms of such a problem will alert the obstetrician in sufficient time to perform a caesarean section before either the mother or the baby get into serious danger.

When deciding whether to suggest to a woman that she has a trial of labour — where labour is allowed to progress naturally but both mother and baby are monitored carefully so a caesarean section can be performed quickly should the need arise — or to recommend an elective caesarean section, the obstetrician has several factors to take into account.

The Reason(s) for the Previous Caesarean Section

The most important factor is why the first caesarean section was performed. This is one reason why it is crucial to talk to your doctor after a caesarean section, so you understand exactly why you needed the operation and to ascertain whether or not you would require caesarean deliveries for future pregnancies.

Some problems which demand a caesarean delivery are unlikely to occur in a subsequent pregnancy and consequently there should not be any reason why you could not have a normal vaginal delivery next time. Placenta praevia and breech position are two such problems that would fall into this non-repeating category. (The exception to this is if you had an abnormality in the shape of your uterine cavity which predisposes a breech position of the baby.)

time, be sure to talk to your obstetrician about this at the antenatal clinic. He or she can then assess whether or not a trial of labour is possible in practical terms and if he or she is prepared to support you in your desire. If the doctor is unwilling to let you try for a vaginal delivery and you are dissatisfied with the reasons given, you can look for another doctor who might hold a different view.

Preparing yourself well during your pregnancy can influence your chances of a successful vaginal delivery. Pay attention to your diet and be rigorous about exercising, so your body is fit and strong for labour. It is also important to attend antenatal classes to brush up on your breathing exercises and relaxation techniques.

I had had an emergency caesarean with my first son because of fetal distress, but I was determined to have a normal birth this time. I had worked really hard at keeping fit during pregnancy and was even swimming ten lengths two days before my labour. My pregnancy went like a dream — no problems at all other than the usual irritations. But I was so nervous when the contractions started — all the talk of a 'trial of labour' made me feel as if I was on trial! Fortunately I had been religiously to NCT classes and had practised my breathing exercises, so I managed to calm myself down. Eight hours from the first contraction I delivered a bouncing baby boy. I have never felt so proud in my life before.

Mary

If you do need a caesarean delivery second time round, then you have the advantage of knowing what to expect and will be able to approach the event with a great deal more confidence and happy anticipation than perhaps you did the first time. You will also know that a caesarean section is not just a life-saving operation without which you and your baby would be severely at risk, but that it is, most important of all, the birth of your child and as such can be a joyful and fulfilling experience to treasure always.

USEFUL
ADDRESSES

Association for Improvements in the Maternity Services
163 Liverpool Road
London N1 0RF
A voluntary organisation campaigning for improvements in the maternity care available in the UK. Can offer advice if you want to try for a vaginal delivery after a caesarean section.

Association of Breastfeeding Mothers
10 Herschell Road
London SE23 1EN
National network of counsellors who can offer advice to breastfeeding mothers.

Association for Post-natal Illness
7 Gowan Avenue
London SW6 6RH
Advice and support offered by mothers who have themselves suffered from postnatal depression, supported by medical experts.

Blisslink
44–5 Museum Street
London WC1A 1LY
Support service for parents with a baby in special care. Set up by BLISS, a charity devoted to raising funds for equipment for SCBUs.

The Compassionate Friends
National Secretary
6 Denmark Street
Bristol BS1 5DQ
International organisation of bereaved parents offering
friendship and support to other parents who have lost a
child of any age.

La Leche League
Box 3424
London WC1 6XX
Help, information and support, plus local groups, for
mothers who are breastfeeding.

MAMA (Meet-a-Mum Association)
3 Woodside Avenue
London SE25
Support for mothers through local contacts.

National Caesarean Support Network
c/o Sheila Tunstall
2 Hurst Park Drive
Huyton
Liverpool L36 1TF
Provides an information service — books, leaflets, etc. —
and a counselling service on a group basis for women who
have had or are about to have a caesarean section delivery.

National Childbirth Trust
9 Queensborough Terrace
London W2 3TB
Runs antenatal classes, which include information on
caesarean sections, and postnatal groups to support new
mothers. Also offers advice on breastfeeding.

NIPPERS
c/o Sam Segal Perinatal Unit
St Mary's Hospital
Praed Street
London W2 1NY
Provides information, advice and parent-to-parent
support groups for parents of premature babies.

Stillbirths and Neonatal Deaths Society
28 Portland Place
London W1N 4DE
Provides support and befriending for parents who have
suffered the loss of a baby around the time of birth.

INDEX

Figures set in *italics* refer to illustrations.